TAKING CARE OF MOTHER, TAKING CARE OF ME

HEYDON BUCHANAN

CLARIOR PRESS

INDIANAPOLIS

Taking Care of Mother, Taking Care of Me.

ISBN: 0-9778140-0-9

Library of Congress Control Number: 2005909441

This book is printed on acid-free paper.

Printed and bound in the United States of America.

This work is based on my personal experiences in caregiving and working with nursing homes, as well as information which other caregivers have shared with me. Further resources are publications and medical research studies which are documented in the notes section at the end of the book. Each caregiving journey is different, and I recommend that caregivers draw on as many sources of helpful information as possible in designing one's own journey; this includes asking the patient's physician about the most current research in methods of treatment. Some peoples' names have been changed or omitted to protect their privacy. Any possible slights against people or institutions are unintentional. Any mistakes contained herein are my own.

DEDICATION

This book is dedicated to

All Family Caregivers

—past, present, and future—

People who understand

Love and Sacrifice

on a higher plane.

A special dedication to

Bernice Ione Foy Buchanan—

a wise, loving, and joyful teacher,

even in her hour of need.

ACKNOWLEDGEMENTS

I wish to acknowledge the following
friends and medical professionals who helped in
some way to make this a better book:
Ann, Carol, Susan, Nancy, Sharon, Stephanie,
Lezlie, Erma, Mirella, Pat, Frances, Mike, and Chris.
My apologies if I've forgotten anyone.

A special acknowledgement to my wife and
fellow caregiver, **Nancy Nienaber Buchanan**,
a very supportive partner throughout, who also always
treated Bernice as lovingly as her own mother.
Thank you, Nancy.

———————————————————————————

Cover designs: Heydon Buchanan
Front cover photo: Nancy Nienaber Buchanan

Table of Contents

CHAPTER 1   COMES A TIME 1
The events one thinks will never happen—
parental death, a disabled widow.

CHAPTER 2   RETURNING Home 8
Changing one's life entirely to fulfill a loving
commitment. The maternal bond in our lives.

CHAPTER 3   THE LIFE WELL-LIVED...................... 13
A special person's life and era. How family and
regional history contributed to this story.
Realizing the need to repay sacrifice.

CHAPTER 4   ARRIVING — HOME IS WHERE THE
HEARTS ARE (1991-1995).................... 54
A young couple meet, fall in love, and make a
good life together. A son returns to the Heartland
and begins parental caregiving. The external
problems of caregiving become evident.

CHAPTER 5   FAMILIES AT THE CROSSROADS 100
A study of family. The very complicated matter
of family dynamics with regard to caregiving for a
parent with Alzheimer's disease. Choosing, or not,
to participate in parental caregiving.

CHAPTER 6   FORGIVENESS 132
Understanding forgiveness. The issue and
importance of forgiveness for caregiver,
care recipient, and other family members.

CHAPTER 7   WORST NIGHTMARE —
THE CATASTROPHIC EFFECT............... 146
The need for caregiver respite. A long, dark,
road trip that brought unknown and unexpected
terror to caregiver and care recipient.

CHAPTER 8   NURSING HOMES —
             A MODERN, SAD REALITY..................163
             The mixed blessing of nursing facilities.
             To end one's life in a nursing home.

CHAPTER 9   NURSING HOMES — ONE, TWO, THREE 180
             A study of three nursing homes. The structure
             of nursing homes. A patient's joy in going
             home from a nursing facility. Helping a loved
             one in a facility with living tools and treats.
             Working with staff.

CHAPTER 10   LOVE AND LAUGHTER 234
             Love and laughter as the most effective
             medications for caregivers and care recipients.
             Unconditional love as gift and reward between
             caregiver and care recipient.

CHAPTER 11   A TIME TO DIE 254
             Facing the end. The price of medical mix-ups
             and administrative errors. The role of hospice
             care in a facility. Sharing the end.

CHAPTER 12   PICKING UP THE PIECES 273
             The shock of loss. Mourning. Duration of grief.

CHAPTER 13   THE FUTURE — ALZHEIMER'S, NURSING
             HOMES, FAMILY CAREGIVING, AND ME 292
             Lessons learned. The national fear of an AD
             diagnosis. The prospect of nursing homes.
             The immense spiritual and financial value of family
             caregivers. The beauty of old age. Moving on.

EPILOGUE 313

NOTES 315

ABOUT THE AUTHOR 318

CHAPTER 1

COMES A TIME…

From delusion lead me to Truth
From darkness lead me to Light
From death lead me to Eternal Life.
  —Hindu prayer from the Sanskrit

One should die proudly when it is no longer possible to
live proudly.
  —Unknown

O N SATURDAY MORNING, JANUARY 12, 1991, I RECEIVED A PHONE
call in Los Angeles (L.A.) from my sister in Indianapolis saying
that our father had just died. Through her tears and shaky voice, I heard
but I didn't hear.

"What? How? What happened?" I asked.

She said that he had been sitting in the chair in his hospital
room while the nurse was straightening up his bed. When the nurse
turned to ask him something, he was gone. Just like that. Just like he
wanted really—here today…gone today….

Dad had been through vascular surgery less than a week before
and had spent several days in intensive care. Then he was transferred to
regular care where he had been for a couple of days. Fortunately, I was
able to speak with him on the phone just when they were transferring
him from intensive care to the regular ward. He had sounded pretty
good.

"Seems like you're healing well," I said.

"Well, I'm much better, but we're not out of the woods yet," he replied.

"Take care. I'll call you soon," I finished, never expecting that that would be our last conversation.

I was in shock about his death, but said I would get a plane for Indianapolis as soon as possible. The next few hours were a blur of slow motion as I made plans and calls to leave work and life in one city and go to a mourning family and funeral preparations in another.

After packing a suitcase, I closed my apartment and caught a cab to Los Angeles International Airport (LAX). The flight was three and a half hours nonstop. It gave me a chance to rest and to absorb the news from the morning.

Dad's death was not a total shock because he was in the hospital, but he was supposedly past the critical part of his recovery. Still, the massive heart attack was a surprise, and beyond that *one's parents just don't die*—a lingering belief from childhood that had stood the test of time. Moreover, this old warrior had survived two major wars among other serious brushes with the grim reaper. He seemed immortal or at least indestructible.

My father had warned me about his impending death. For the last dozen years, during my annual vacation to Indianapolis, Dad had made sure I knew that death would be there for him any time. By the second evening of each vacation, he and I would stay up late talking, and he would start, "You know, with the condition of my heart...." Then he would move on to "And the papers are upstairs in my metal box. The obituary is written. The burial instructions have been completed. There's a list of people to notify. I would like to have 'Amazing Grace' sung and...." And so on. Twelve years of trial runs, and now it had happened.

Beyond the actual death, I reflected on the more current preoccupation of his last fifteen months—trying to convince me to move back to Indianapolis. As his health declined, and more importantly, as the disability of his caregiver—my mother—increased, he became more persistent in his requests for me to return home. Dad wanted me to take care of him and Mother. Since I was single and without dependents, he felt comfortable asking that. Mother would never ask nor expect it.

In our transcontinental telephone conversations, my father often brought up "Mother's memory problem." He was becoming increasingly distressed. After all, when the person who takes care of you is suddenly in need of care herself, it's a threatening situation—particularly when her condition seems to be chronic and progressive.

However, I believe he also wanted more time for the two of us to talk before he died. I called home weekly, and we spoke a lot during my annual vacation there, but he wanted to talk more. There was really no one else for him to speak with on some matters.

One thing was certain: he knew that Mother's memory problem was beyond simple forgetfulness, and it was also beyond his ability to help her. He was also concerned about Mother's welfare if he should die first.

In addition to our weekly phone calls, I also corresponded with my parents through letters. Mother would handwrite letters since her handwriting was very clear and precise. Dad was more comfortable with a typewriter because his handwriting looked like that of most doctors—illegible. During the last couple years of his life, he had some tremors from a transient ischemic attack (TIA) so even the typewriter became too difficult to use. Subsequently, I bought him a cassette recorder and taught him how to use it, so our supplemental correspondence was through cassette tapes.

Not long before he died, I received a tape with his thoughts and sentiments on various topics. Much of it was identifying details in photographs from his professional life that were hanging in his office. Also, he included his wishes for what he would like for me to do in caring for Mother. He said, "You know that the only responsibility I'm placing on you is to insure your mother's welfare in the future. She's going to need someone to lean on, and that is a responsibility that I have to put in your hands. And lastly, of course you know I love you. Dad." After a pause, he added in a somber voice, "There is one final thought. In case of my demise, which is certainly inevitable, I do not want your mother to be placed in a nursing home. I've been in a number of those homes, and it's no place to be." Amen, but my father had no grasp of what caregiving entailed. What he did have was a strong sense of responsibility, loyalty, and mostly unspoken love.

Like many men, my father had trouble verbalizing emotions of affection. So, having that tape with his expression "I love you" is unusual—not only the sentiment but having it in his voice. His request that

I take care of Mother was not necessary since I didn't need a push or reminder from anyone to do that.

*****

In June 1990, seven months before Dad passed away, my parents had flown to L.A. to visit me. As Dad and I were walking one night after dinner, I was surprised to see that he could walk no more than a block without having to stop and rest. This was a man who had been in good physical shape until a few years before, and equally important, a person with a pretty strong heart. Now, however, his arteries were truly rebelling, having been stockpiled with the residual effects of smoking and excess cholesterol. While we stopped to rest for a moment, Dad asked again about my coming home, mentioning his condition and Mother's. I told him I was thinking about it.

He also told me that in my absence from Indianapolis he had chosen one of my four sisters to be Power of Attorney (POA). I agreed with his choice. At that stage of my parents' lives, a POA would basically just pay their monthly bills. Dad was projecting a faster advancing of the dementia than was actually happening, probably due to his fear; subsequently, he designated the POA, and I don't know whether he consulted with Mother on the whole action or not. A couple of years after that, Mother told me she wanted to control the money instead of having a POA. I reminded her of Dad's action. She said, "I don't like that. Dad did that to me all my life." I believe such male control of the checkbook was especially true of their generation. I really didn't want to be POA as well as primary caregiver. The POA duty didn't take much time, but for the primary caregiver it would have been just one more task on top of the others.

Mother's desire to control her own money was understandable on an additional level as well. Alzheimer's patients often feel that they are losing control of their lives, or that someone is taking that control away from them. For some patients, there is a strong feeling that their things—possessions, money, etc.—are being stolen from them. This was not much of a complaint from Bernice, though there were two instances when family members visited the townhouse, and she told me afterwards that she thought one of them had taken a particular thing. Mother may have been right, but it involved pieces of jewelry, and I wouldn't have known if some piece was missing or not. I have read of some Alzheimer's patients commonly complaining of things being taken. In some cases, the suspicions of the AD patient are quite justified when relatives move quickly to take a person's things away; that is, after the patient has been diagnosed but is still living in his or her own home.

*****

In September, three months later, I visited Indianapolis to see the progression of Mother's and Dad's health. Mother did well in masking her forgetfulness and acted as though her forgetting was a very little matter. She also thought her memory lapses were a normal part of aging and didn't want me to worry about it. It was again apparent that Dad was becoming more limited in physical endurance, and subsequently his doctor was strongly recommending vascular surgery.

After a week's stay, I returned to Los Angeles. During the next month, I decided to move back to Indianapolis. There was no doubt that I should help my parents in whatever way I could, and that help would not be possible by long distance. The potential scenario that worried me most was if Dad should become disabled and need more care from Mother. This would undoubtedly aggravate her condition, and the falling domino effect could be disastrous.

In November I told Dad of my decision. He, in turn, scheduled his surgery for after New Year's Day. There were a number of personal and professional details to closing my life in Los Angeles, and I had slowly begun the process as Thanksgiving approached. I was in that process when the fateful phone call came in January telling me of his death.

*****

A friend picked me up at the Indianapolis airport, and we went to my folks' home. Mother was composed and doing well, in spite of the death of her mate of fifty-three years. They had left nothing unsaid as far as I knew. She was calm but a bit confused. I learned later that this was one of those traumatic events that can suddenly spike a slowly-progressive dementia condition such as Alzheimer's disease.

Later, we went through the funeral preparations at the mortuary. The service and burial were set for Wednesday, January 16th. As we waited for the day of the funeral, I noticed some of Mother's forgetfulness but didn't try to examine it. The loss of my father and all that entailed were more than enough for me to digest until after the funeral.

We had the viewing and reception at the mortuary on Tuesday evening. Many people came by to pay respects and share remembrances. This was "The Colonel." He had touched a lot of lives, and through friendship and community service, he had left an indelible print. In manner and action, he was one of a kind.

On the day of the funeral, we had a memorial service at the mortuary prior to the burial service. A number of us spoke about his effect on us. The funeral was everything Dad had wanted. Many people whose lives he had affected gathered together to remember and bury him. There was a military honor guard and a twenty-one-gun salute. It was a cold, rainy day in Crown Hill Cemetery when we buried him, and the process had all the ceremony he would have loved.

After the burial, I had three days left before I had to be back at work in Los Angeles—three days to evaluate Mother's condition and discuss it with my siblings. After those three days, there was really no doubt about it—Mother shouldn't be living alone for long. The loss of her spouse, plus the increasing disability, made her vulnerability more and more apparent.

Mother's forgetting had begun not long after her knee replacement surgery in early 1988. She had had general anesthesia, and from what medical research has now learned, that may well have initiated the memory problems. Her best friend in Indianapolis first noticed Mother's problem with memory after the surgery. I'll call her friend Selma. Selma was very astute in such observations; there was no problem with Selma's memory, or mental functioning since she was still playing tournament bridge.

Again, I confirmed my decision. I would wrap up things in Los Angeles as soon as possible and return to Indianapolis to live with Mother. Mother was, as usual, not requesting any change in my life to accommodate hers.

Quite seriously and considerately she said, "Heydon, I'll be all right. I don't want you to change your whole life just for me."

"I know," I answered, "but, it's my choice, and that's what I want to do."

Mother was sincere and confident and said that she would get by on her own. That being said, she was happy that I was moving back if that was what I really wanted to do. Further, she said she'd be glad since she didn't want to live alone. That was a difference between her and Dad—he didn't hesitate to ask me to come back, while she truly wouldn't ask me to change my life just to help her, no matter what her condition.

One thing I knew for sure—I wouldn't be comfortable with her living alone at this time, and probably from here on out. Long distance worry would keep my head and heart in Indianapolis, so it made sense to move back. The family was in agreement. My sisters would keep watch over Mother until my permanent return in six or seven weeks.

We said good-bye, and I left for the airport. The flight back to Los Angeles gave me plenty of time to think. Now it was not just absorbing my father's death; it was closing my life in L.A., moving back to Indianapolis, and making a plan which would allow me to carry out this new responsibility—taking care of Mother. It had been a long week, yet the serious life changes were really just beginning.

CHAPTER 2

RETURNING HOME

Our sweetest experiences of affection are meant to point
us to that realm which is the real and endless home of the
heart.
　—Henry Ward Beecher

Love doesn't hide. It stays and fights. It goes the distance,
that's why love is so strong. So it can carry you all the way
home.
　—Unknown

I WOKE UP AS THE PLANE TOUCHED DOWN IN LOS ANGELES. COMING
out of sleep, I wondered about the recent events. Was last week real?
Did all of that truly happen? Was my father dead? Was my mother in the
early phase of dementia? Was I giving up my home here and moving
back to Indianapolis? Before the plane got to the terminal, I remembered that it was all quite real.

*****

So I began the process of closing down my life in L.A. Being
single and without children made my decisions and actions much simpler than they would have been otherwise. Yet leaving home, work, and
friends required a lot of time and effort.

My apartment was in Hollywood, about a mile from work—a
simple commute compared to most Angelenos. The easy part of that
closing was to simply give a month's notice when I knew the departure
date. The more difficult portion was handling the furniture and other

possessions—some went to storage, some were shipped, and other things were given away.

Leaving work was not so difficult due to the current state of the graphics business. Advertising typography—the specialty of our studio—was in a state of transition as it went from using mainframe computers to personal computers. The shop was slow to change in technology and subsequently was losing some big accounts. Someone would have been laid off before long. It wouldn't have been me since I ranked high in seniority, but it would have been a young guy with a family. So, I volunteered for the layoff, and that worked for everyone.

I didn't like giving up the good income, as well as the opportunity to retrain on new equipment and stay current in the industry; however, I had made my decision. There was a sad part to leaving coworkers who had become friends, but fortunately the shop was not left in a bad position.

Concerning friends outside of work, we said our good-byes and made our plans to stay in touch. As I drove away from Los Angeles, the one constant thought in my mind was that the work I was going toward was far more important than the job I was leaving behind.

*****

If in any way I've implied that my decision to return to Indianapolis was difficult, that was not the case at all. Since Dad tended to exaggerate and overreact in his later years, I just had to take some time to evaluate the immediacy of their need for me to be there for caregiving. I knew that he was becoming more physically limited, but figured that maybe my sisters could help with what errands might come up. After seeing his condition in June 1990, I knew that the old warrior was truly deteriorating.

Now, since Dad had suddenly died, and Mother was left alone with her memory problem, I had absolutely no hesitation in choosing to move back and help her in whatever way I could. I did not think of it as a sacrifice in any way. Simply put, if I hadn't moved back to take care of her, I couldn't have lived with myself.

My life in Los Angeles was pleasant, and I enjoyed friends and the Southern California lifestyle, especially being close to the beach. I was able to do some volunteer work, so my life didn't seem so self-centered. However, that life paled in value when compared with the possibility of helping my mother through this most difficult period of her life. Not only was she my mother and the person who had done more for me than anyone else on earth, she was also the kindest and finest person I'd ever known.

On hearing my news of leaving, a friend in L.A. somewhat jokingly said, "I can understand that you want to help your mother, but to actually live with her?"

"Well," I replied, "if my mother was difficult, I'd still feel responsible for her, but I wouldn't live with her. Sanity is too precious for that. But Mother is quite the opposite of difficult. She's a gentle, loving, and considerate person who benefits everyone she comes in contact with."

How can we not take care of our parents in their hour of need? This especially applies to a Mother—the symbol of what's right with the world. A Mother may be the most sacred symbol of all in this life. It's no wonder that matriarchy was the rule of order in some past societies, before we moved into the realm of might makes right. In a moment of critical need, we call for the person who has cared for and comforted us most throughout. Countless soldiers who have fallen with mortal combat wounds have called out for "Mother." This final desperate cry for help is made to the person who comforted them when all others failed. Our mother is one of the principal people, if not the first, that we would die for.

*****

The biggest puzzle about life seems to be the first one we encounter. On entry into this world, the shock of light and coldness leave us stunned. Without intellect, we ask, "Where am I? Why is it so cold? Why is it so bright?"

Soon after, we are cleaned and cuddled and fed. Then, part of the fear and discomfort go away as we are comforted—comforted with warmth and food, later to be augmented by the security of love. The most consistent provider of that love is usually our mother. Subsequently, a bond begins between the provider and the child—a bond of dependence that evolves into a higher level, one of appreciation and gratitude. Some call it love. In the world of give and take, the Mother gives and the child takes.

Following adolescence, this family relationship could end completely, and the world would still go around. However, something much larger would die—we would lose access to the love and wisdom of the person who delivered us into this world; we would lose knowledge of ancestors and family history; we would lose the person most likely to care whether we live or die. In fact, instead of ending, the mother-child relationship just changes to another level. After leaving home, the adult moves on to develop his or her separate life away from the parental structure.

The spirit of love—in this case maternal love—is a force that allows us to keep and bolster our humanity. Without respect for the institution of Motherhood and other similar humanitarian efforts, man could easily destroy himself physically, mentally, emotionally, and spiritually in any number of self-destructive pursuits.

As our parents age and face increasing disabilities, we are reminded once again of that earlier dependent relationship. The roles are about to be reversed. Our help is greatly needed. It's time for the child to give and the parent to take—a natural progression in the cycle of life. A couple of relevant examples come to mind.

A classic Japanese film, *The Ballad of Narayama*,[1] demonstrates the suffering of old age as well as a parent-child bond in later years. In that case, it shows the Mother-son relationship. Based on an ancient Japanese legend, the setting is a small mountain village in times past. There is a perpetual shortage of food, so when a person reaches age seventy, he or she must leave the village and ascend Mt. Narayama to the dying grounds where they wait alone for death. The principal character is a grandmother about to turn seventy. She has led an exemplary life and is cheerfully ready to accept her fate. Her son tries to accept the tradition but is very distraught as the time approaches. He tries to convince her to stay in the village one more year. She says no and accepts the tradition in order to continue setting an example for all. He carries her on his back most of the way up the mountain, and his pleas to change her mind increase as they ascend. She stops talking along the way in order to mentally detach herself from the living. The story shows the anguish of a loving son as he has to say goodbye to his mother for the last time. In the style of Kabuki Theater, a woman sings mournfully in the background, "The bonds linking a Mother and son are interwoven like finespun yarn.... For this kind and loving Mother comes the day of fated parting. Where could a Mother's son be who writhes not on such a day?" It is very poignant and well depicts the pain of losing your oldest friend, teacher, and advocate.

Another example of the Mother-son bond and separation is seen from the view of the Mother's anguish. In the authorized biography of Mother Teresa by Kathryn Spink,[2] the author writes, "The story of how she rescued a woman who had been left to die on the streets of Calcutta was one which Mother Teresa would afterwards tell to audiences throughout the world. What caused that woman to weep, she informed them, was not the fact that she was half-consumed by maggots and on the point of death, but that the person who had deserted her was her son, that she was alone and unwanted even by her own family."

I don't believe there's any way to minimize the emotional pain of the son in the first example, or the Mother in the second. They are both cases of true human pathos.

*****

Now it's time to talk about my experience in this realm. This story is about my opportunity to help my mother as she became increasingly and totally dependent on others. It is also the story of her journey through Shakespeare's seven ages of man, and how we faced those final challenges together.

I had no idea how long this caregiving would last. I had no idea how much it would cost. I had no concept of how hard it would be. I had not the slightest clue of what family problems lay ahead. And, I had not even imagined the great spiritual dividends I would receive when all was said and done. What I did know was that it was the right thing to do. The joys, as well as the trials and tribulations, lay straight ahead.

CHAPTER 3

THE LIFE WELL-LIVED

Living by example is not the main thing in influencing others, it is the only thing.
—Albert Schweitzer

As I drove into Arizona and left California behind, I began to think of my mother's life—her life in its entirety—life beyond her children who always called for her attention, who always needed something from her.

When we reflect on a Mother's life, it's easy to see how selfish and self-centered children can be. Kids all too often view their mother as someone who was born simply to take care of their needs. In early years, they may even consider their mother to be one of generic issue; that is, one Mother being the same as another. However, once they spend some time around the parents of their friends, they have a chance to see the difference in styles of parenting and the difference in temperament and demeanor from their own Mother and Father.

Bernice Buchanan was not simply a remarkable Mother, though that qualification in itself would rate her quite highly. She was also a remarkable person—a person who had known and spread joy and love from her very early days on. Mother set an example of how a conscious, conscientious, productive, joyful, loving life is lived. She walked the talk, but she never talked it, except to her kids since we needed direction while growing up. She taught by example. She never preached nor drew attention to herself. She never smoked nor drank nor yelled nor used profanity nor spoke badly of anyone else, nor was she ever a hypocrite. She was a role model.

Bernice loved going to church, but she never insisted that anyone else go—except for her children who had to go to Sunday school, and that was a joint decision with Dad. She really didn't care which religion people had or which church or temple they went to, or whether they had or professed any religion at all. She cared about each person as an individual, and believed that God loved each person. What concerned her was the end product. To be a regular part of her life, someone would have to be a friendly and honest person who treated other people well.

Her children were raised with the unwritten rule of honesty. I don't remember the specific lesson my parents used to stress the importance of honesty any more than I remember some examples for other principles our parents instilled in us; however, the lesson was something that stuck. I know there must have been verbal admonitions about honesty and its rightness, but I don't remember the exact illustrations.

The verbal training I do remember came when it was appropriate to the situation at hand. For example, if one of us said something negative to a sibling or about another person, Mother would say, "If you can't say something nice, don't say anything at all." When we got into some childhood argument, we were separated, sent to our rooms and told, "If you can't play together nicely, then you can't play together."

Another principle I remember was, "Do unto others, as you would have them do unto you." That one came my way after I was in a fight at school one day. It happened at recess, and I don't believe it even got reported. There was a known bully who wanted to intimidate me, probably since I was the new kid in school. He started pushing me around; I hit him and knocked him down. The other guys there put me on their shoulders and were carrying me around and cheering. Maybe they figured his power was broken. After school I walked home and found Mother ironing. When I walked in the house, she asked how school went, and I told her everything. She frowned about the incident, and soon came out with "Do unto others...."

I quickly replied, "Well, he hit me first, so I hit him back. He did unto me, so I did unto him."

"That's not how it works," she said. "Do you feel better after what you did?"

I waited for a moment. "Not really," I replied.

"Maybe you should call him, see how he's doing," she added.

"I don't know about that," I said. However, in a few minutes I had found and dialed his number. A boy answered.

"Billy?" I asked.

"Yes?" he replied.

"This is Heydon—from school."

Silence on the other phone.

"I just wanted to say I'm sorry about hitting you today."

Still a pause—finally, "Oh that's okay. It didn't hurt, not much...." He sounded like he was simulating a faint.

"Well, okay, I'll see you tomorrow," I replied.

"Hey," Billy answered, "do you want to come over and play football?" He may have wanted a chance to get back at me.

"Okay, if it's all right with Mother, and I can get a ride."

Mother said fine, drove me over to Billy's house, and we played one-man teams against each other. It was fulfilling to run full-speed and tackle one another, and we were exhausted at the end. He and I became pretty good friends and went on to play football together in junior high school.

In retrospect, I see in that particular situation that Mother was thinking *proactive* while I was thinking *reactive*. In that case, her "Do unto others...." was really an offshoot of the principle "Turn the other cheek." It's a very idealistic approach, and few people are able to carry that one out completely. Essentially, it was a struggle of "An eye for an eye" versus "Turn the other cheek." It may be especially appropriate to mention that example here since the world's ongoing hotspots seem to be hung up on "An eye for an eye" or in practice "Two eyes for an eye." Mother's lesson never took complete hold with me, as I seemed to be about halfway between the two philosophies. So, Dad gave me a few boxing lessons. I still got into some fights but only as a last resort. Mother lived every principle she advocated to us children. She never retaliated for pain done to her by others. She never passed on pain to someone else, except God perhaps.

My parents were very idealistic. They really lived on a higher plane of conduct and simply did their best. Both were raised in the tradition of service to others, and belief in the inherent value of all humanity. They didn't live in an ivory tower nor lead sheltered lives. Both had been tested in numerous ways, by the Depression for one instance.

Dad was also quite a warrior, and that role had started early in his life. He fought a lot as a kid. He grew up in a tough neighborhood in tough times where fighting was rarely an option. He told me he had to fight his way home from school most every day. Then he took his fighting to the boxing ring and won the Golden Gloves.

My parents had no tolerance for prejudice. They were highly principled and had been from the time their union was formed—when they were college students and falling in love. We were raised in that environment. I've never heard a hurtful racial or religious remark from my sisters, and I don't believe I have used one either. Whenever we came in contact with other people—different color, religion, shape, size, nationality, age, etc.—we just addressed the person as a fellow human being. No doubt we had personal thoughts about some people—for example, someone being verbally obnoxious—but we usually kept them to ourselves. We had lived in the South and in the North, and we encountered as much prejudice up North as we had down South.

Actually, I do remember one case of using a racial slur. It was in late December, 1953. We lived in Tampa, Florida, and had gone to Indianapolis, Indiana, to spend Christmas with my father's sister and her husband. Dad had recently returned from the Korean War, so the trip north was something of a reunion for that as well. We kids hadn't been North before, so we were very excited to see and play in the snow.

On the return trip to Tampa, we kids riding in the back got into an argument. My twin sisters were five-years-old, and I was seven. In the heat of an argument—and probably desperate for an insult—one of us (probably me) said, "You're a n _ _ _ _ _ ." We were driving on a two-lane highway—there were no interstates then—about 50 mph. My parents both looked at each other in shock, and my father immediately pulled over to the side of the highway and stopped.

Mother and Dad turned to us in the back seat and Dad asked angrily, "What did you say?" We didn't answer.

"Where did you hear that word? That's a bad word. Don't ever say it again!"

"Well," I answered, "Aunt _ _ _ _ _ and Uncle _ _ _ said it." This was true, and I was hoping it might lighten his anger. It didn't.

"That doesn't make it right! That's just plain ignorance to use that word," he replied. That was a big statement for him to make. That aunt was his only sister, someone he loved very much, and they had been through a lot together. Still, he and Mother wouldn't put up with that language, or the feelings it represented.

Concerning profanity, I rarely even heard the word "damn" from him and never in Mother's presence. Once I saw him driving in a nail to repair something when he suddenly banged his finger hard. His face grimaced in pain, and he said, "Da…" stopping as he saw Mother's face, and then finishing as "Darn." They had both agreed long ago on the atmosphere they wanted in their home. My father had been around plenty of profanity, as most men have. He was a soldier for many years and heard plenty of it in the army. The officers with whom he served would not often use it. An exception to that rule in the high command was General Patton; profanity was a large part of his vocabulary. Dad knew him but didn't really care for his style because Patton was egotistical, ostentatious with his pearl-handled revolvers, and very profane.

In World War II (WWII), Dad was often called Buck by friends, as he had been earlier in life. He had many close brushes with death; the first was before he even officially got into combat. His transport ship to North Africa from Scotland—the SS Strathallan—was torpedoed and sunk. The ship was carrying a reported 6,000 allied soldiers plus a lot of nurses, principally Scottish nurses. He survived after finally jumping overboard and then staying in the water overnight holding onto a piece of flotsam. He was picked up with others the next day, taken to Algiers and then joined the combat movement across North Africa, then Sicily, and all the Italian campaign.

During WWII, he also saw prejudice in the military time and again against Blacks, American Indians, and Japanese-American soldiers. He had little patience for that. The stupidity of prejudice in general, but especially among troops fighting a common enemy, was maddening for him to witness. Not only were lower rank soldiers prejudiced, but some officers at all levels held the prejudice too.

Buck had an official army photo of the famed Japanese-American unit—the 442nd Regimental Combat Team—as they were being reviewed by General Mark Clark and then Secretary of the Navy, James Forrestall, during a stop in Italy. Dad was very impressed with the bravery of the 442nd, as they had the highest number of purple hearts of any unit in the army, as well as a high number of other awards, and those represented a great deal of courage and service.

After WWII, Buck stayed in service and went on to another war in Korea, surviving that one as well. His metal had been tested and not by some textbook adventure. Korea had probably taken him over the edge, and the wounds of war were soon to start taking their due. However, regardless of all the danger and stress he had experienced, and all the brutality of one nation toward another that he had witnessed, he still held very high standards about how life should be lived—with respect for all human beings and just treatment for everyone.

My father loved poetry and other fine literature, as well as a variety of classical music. He read poetry to us as we were growing up, and he was most animated in his presentations—sad when the subject called for it, and full of laughter when it was funny. His favorite book for reading to us was *A Treasury of the Familiar*—an anthology of classic poetry, essays, Bible chapters and verses, anthems, anonymous musings, and on and on. Comprised of literature, philosophy, and wisdom from around the world, it was a remarkable collection. He told me more than once, "If you read this book from cover to cover, you've had an education."

We kids loved to see Dad feel good. I suppose that was because it kept his depression at bay. He and Mother enjoyed the big band sound, and they had fun dancing as well. On some Sunday afternoons in Tampa, we would go out to the Officer's Club at MacDill Air Force Base. After swimming during the afternoon, the family would have supper. Then the kids watched TV with all the other kids there while Mother and Dad went to the dance floor. They were fun times.

Our parents were dedicated not only to their family but also to the local community and the nation as a whole. Their lives could be defined as those of service to others. They had a heavy sense of responsibility to try and make things right for everyone. I remember a number of times when Dad said to me, "If a person doesn't do something to make a better world, he or she has lived a wasted life." He practiced that intensely, putting a lot of pressure on himself and those of us close to him.

At my father's funeral, we had a memorial service where people could speak of their relationship with him and whatever effect he had had on them. After I spoke of his effect on me, I added an appreciation for his foresight in choosing Mother as his partner for life. Further, his choice of mates was also one of the smartest moves he had made—not only for his children but for himself; otherwise, the intensity of his energy and drive would have destroyed him early on without the essential, calming nature of Mother. She was the tranquil, sturdy base that made it all possible. In that vein, she probably saved the lives of us children as well, for if we had continued at the pace he maintained, we would surely have burned out early.

Neither of our parents seemed to really fear much of anything, though Dad had an underlying worry about poverty—a carryover from the Depression. Each parent had incredible strength of purpose yet very different energy. For Dad, it was more a "man's driving strength" that carried him through. For Mother, it was her faith and serenity and joy in living life. They both believed in the health of happy laughter and also in doing the right thing.

Following his funeral, we sent out a thank you card to those who attended and those who sent cards or made a donation to their church's soup kitchen where we had requested donations be sent. On the front of the card I designed and composed, I borrowed a line from Mr. Shakespeare as a fitting epitaph—"He was a man, take him all in all. We shall not see his like again." The same could equally be said for Mother except that she was able to live on an even higher plane, part of which was facilitated by Dad's outside labor; we were fortunate to have a stay-at-home Mother. They were a unique couple who did their best throughout their lives, and then passed on to the next life. I mention my parents' individual lives and their life together because it is an important portion of my mother's whole life; and that is the purpose of this chapter.

Before moving into the story of the effect of Alzheimer's disease (AD) on one victim—my mother, Bernice Buchanan—it is important to see her whole life, her unique and pure humanity. When many people see an Alzheimer's victim, or simply hear the dreaded words Alzheimer's disease, they can't see beyond the devastation of the victim—the horror of mental and physical disintegration which only get worse in this terminal illness. It is fearful; however, it is more important to recognize the humanity of the victim, before and during the progression of this illness. It is important to realize that not all people respond alike as the illness grabs hold of them. Their response and reactions can be linked to their inherent nature, their faith, how they've lived their life, how they've been treated, how effective their support system is, and probably other things that I don't know about.

What I do know is that the most effective contribution I made in helping Mother was my portion of the love we shared during the struggles with the disease. What I also realized was that she was a true teacher through the end since she also showed me what a good death is like.

In speaking of our joint trip through Alzheimer's, I tell people that I handled the outer problems while Mother kept the inner problems at bay. Together we made it. Whether in her earlier healthy years, or when facing the challenge of a tough and terminal foe, she continued to serve as a teacher, giving of herself until the end. I would simply say she was my guru, and I thank God that I was given such a great Mother and teacher.

Bernice's evaluation of people included the concept of good guys and bad guys. Those terms came from the era in which she grew up. I never heard her use the term "bad guy"; however, if she liked and respected a man, she would smile and say, "He's a good guy." Another standard of her evaluation would be between people who are nice and those who are mean; or those who love and those who live without it. I've seen her interacting with rich people and poor, and that didn't alter her demeanor in either case. She was consistent; she was real; she was joyful; and most all people enjoy those traits in a fellow human being.

Mother appreciated simple honesty, affection, sincerity, and a sense of humor. Kermit the Frog sat in a chair near her sewing table, so she always had a friend at hand. I should add here that in later years at the nursing home when I would tuck Mother in to sleep, I also put Kermit's head next to hers on the pillow. It was a precious scene, and I believe it gave her some comfort and a little sense of security, so she wouldn't feel so alone in the dark.

Now, let's take a look at Bernice's whole life. Through her early scrapbook and notes, her accounts, those of other family members, and other people who knew her and were affected by her, I have pieced together this history.

*****

This is the life of a person who was born in a mythic era and area of America. She was born and raised in Indiana, a state in the fabled Heartland. Further, Indiana is essentially by location and tradition—at least as portrayed in many movies—the Heart of the Heartland. Since Mother's time on earth could best be defined as a life of love, I think of her as the Heart of the Heart of the Heartland. To my perception, and that of others with their own description, she walked in the Grace of God.

The basic character of Heartlanders is known nationwide as amiable, hospitable, simple, honest, and considerate. It was from this region and foundation that Abraham Lincoln came and then gained national recognition. No doubt the finest personal contribution from the Heartland to the nation was Abraham Lincoln—a rare jewel.

A more recent example of a popular politician from this area was President Ronald Reagan. His image and demeanor conveyed trust. I won't get into his politics, but his childhood home deserves a note here since it was relevant to his charm and this story. Ronald Reagan was born in Tampico, Illinois, a very small farm town in the northwestern portion of the state. Tampico is also where my mother's family—the Foys—had lived since the early 1850s.

Daniel Foy—Bernice's great-grandfather—was one of the first half-dozen settlers to come to Tampico. A pioneer in that rolling prairie land, Daniel arrived in Tampico in 1854, migrating from Cattaraugus County, New York. He had first created a settlement close to Tampico in the Prophetstown Township in 1847 before moving over to Tampico. Daniel was born July 31, 1822, in Napoli, New York. His father, William Foy, born in 1788, and mother, Ruth Morrell Foy, born in 1790, were natives of Vermont. Daniel Foy was the first elected supervisor of Tampico Township and served for two years from 1861-63. He was too old to serve in the Union Army during the Civil War, but I've read that Tampico did send their "quota" of soldiers to serve in the "war of the rebellion." Daniel's nephew, Charles E. Foy, served in the Union Army; he enlisted in the 34th Illinois Volunteer Infantry and participated in all his regiment's engagements. Daniel and Matilda (Williams) Foy had a large family with their nine children. Daniel died in 1899, and Matilda (1821-1911) survived him by twelve years. Birthing all those children, she still lived to the age of ninety in a harsh environment—the strong constitution of pioneers.

Daniel and Matilda's son, Milton (1855-1937), also a farmer, was my mother's paternal grandfather. Mother remembered him as a very quiet and serious man. A photo of Milton with Bernice and her brother Bernard in 1916 shows Milton as a lean, somber fellow with a drooping moustache. Little Bernard also looked serious, in line with his grandfather's appearance. However, at age three, Mother had already developed her classic bright smile.

An important addition to the family was Milton's wife, Charlotte (Pet) Van Drew Foy (1863-1946), Mother's paternal grandmother and a major influence on Bernice's life. Pet was descended from the Pennsylvania Dutch. From Grandma Pet, Bernice received love, laughter and a devotion to work; and most importantly—working joyfully. Many a time from my childhood on, Mother and I would be sharing a laugh about something, and she would say, "Oh, I wish you could have known Grandma Pet. She was so much fun!" Grandma Pet died the year I was born. I have a photo of her during Mother's childhood, and Pet did have a great smile—a photographic smile quite atypical of the staid image portrayed by the farm couple in the classic Grant Wood 1930 painting *American Gothic*. On the other hand, Pet's husband Milton appeared as somber as the man in that painting. From what I've read and heard, Grandma Pet was quite exceptional in that pioneer farm town. I have included a photo of her with two small boys that illustrates her happy nature. She's probably one of so many unsung heroines who have made this a better country and world. She kept a smile on her face, joy in her heart, and a *can-do* attitude.

Milton and Pet had only one child—their son, Louis Calvin Foy (1884-1949). That was Bernice's father and my maternal grandfather. Grandma Pet spent much time with Bernice and other children, and she was much-loved by all of them. My ninety-year-old Aunt Evelyn, who was married to Bernice's brother, Bernard, confirmed this not long ago.

Aunt Evelyn went on to tell me that Grandma Pet feared a bit for Bernice's future—that Bernice may be hurt since she was so nice and trusting. It's true that Mother kept that trust in people and by combining that trust with her own intuition, she could judge a person's heart and character when she met them. Like Bernice, I've always felt it's important

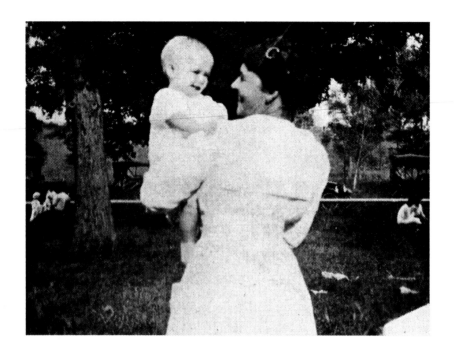

Bernice Ione Foy, 1913— Merom, Indiana
A smiling baby en route to becoming a happy child

1913   1914—No privacy for her bath

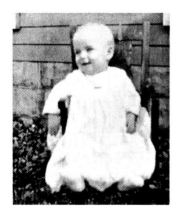
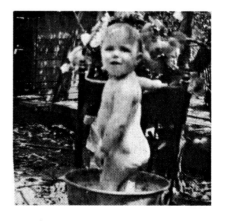

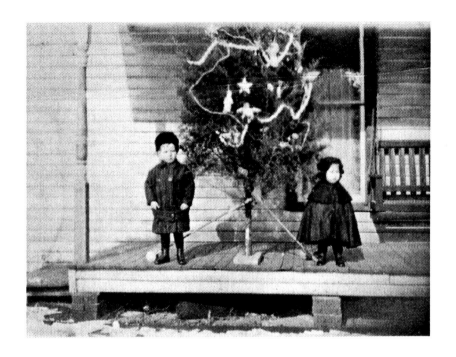

Bernard and Bernice, Christmas, 1915—Merom, Indiana

1917—Bicknell, Indiana

Bernice, Bernard
& Grandpa Milton

Bernice, Bernard &
James David (friend)

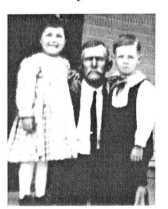

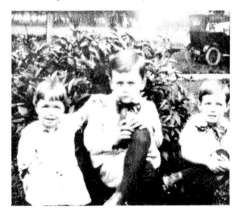

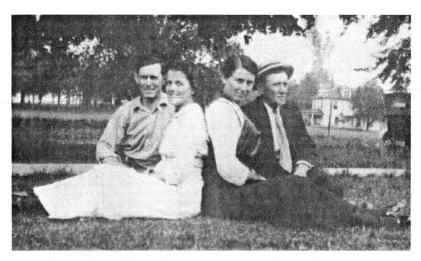

Left: Louis and Bessie Foy (Bernice & Bernard's parents)
(with two friends, on the right), circa 1905— Tampico, Illinois

Below: Bernice, first row on the left; Bernard, last row, on right
Bernice's 4th birthday party, April 12, 1917— Bicknell, Indiana

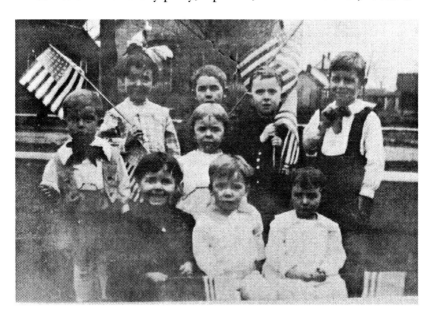

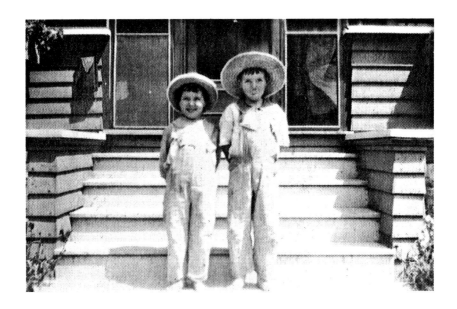

Bernice & Bernard, circa 1919, Bicknell, Indiana

Grandma Pet with
two friends

Bernard, Robert &
Bernice Foy, circa 1920

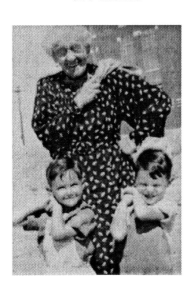

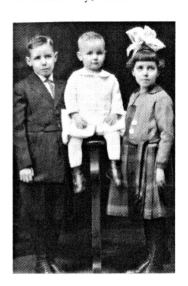

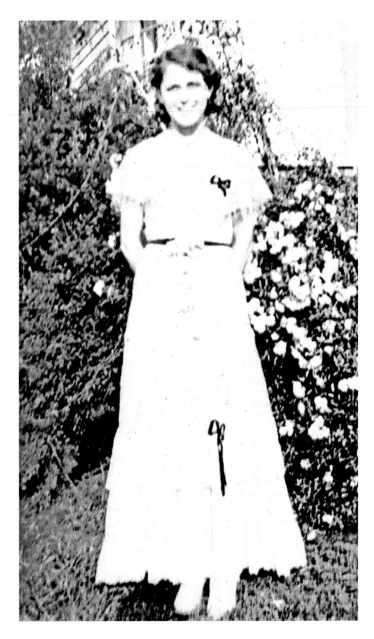

Bernice on High School Graduation Day, 1931,
Bloomington High School, Bloomington, Indiana
(Class Valedictorian was Ross Lockridge, Jr.,
author of *Raintree County*.)

to give everyone a chance. I believe it brings out the best in someone when they know that you trust them. By doing this, you can avoid pre-judging someone—in essence, avoiding prejudice.

As my grandfather grew up, he knew that he didn't want to stay in farming as his father had. Louis was interested in wood—all types of wood. He developed great skill in carving and doing inlaid work, but that was really more of an avocation for him. He became involved in the lumber business, and that is where he spent the rest of his working life—first as a salesman, then as lumberyard manager, then as co-owner. With increasing opportunities, he moved from one town and lumber-yard to another. Louis married Bessie Blanche Darnell (1887-1950), and they moved to Merom, Indiana in 1910 where he managed a lumberyard.

Merom is Indiana's highest point on the Wabash River, which separates Indiana from Illinois. Merom Bluffs is 200 feet above the river and has a very scenic view extending beyond the river to Illinois. Over the centuries it had been used by Native Americans, and the evidence of their occupancy is recorded in the Indian burial mounds nearby. William Henry Harrison built a hospital camp there in 1811 as he passed through en route to Tippecanoe and American history. Merom was laid out and established by 1817 and had hopes of becoming a major city. In 1819, Merom became the Sullivan County Seat. The town was a hub of Wa-bash River traffic and trade. Similar to Tom Sawyer's Hannibal, Mis-souri, Merom's prominence had depended greatly on the river. There was pressure to centralize the County Seat, so Merom lost that position in 1842. Then the railroad and main highway passed Merom by, and the town stayed locked in time—an isolated model of early Americana.

Louis and Bessie's first son, Bernard, was born in Merom in 1911. Then their only daughter, Bernice, was born there in 1913. In 1916 the family left Merom with better opportunity for Louis in the management of another lumber company in Bicknell, Indiana, thirty miles away. Bicknell was founded in 1875, and its principal industry was bituminous coal. It was in Bicknell that the two young Foys found their closest childhood friends. Both Bernice and Bernard told me of the joy of those friendships that they recalled with great fondness.

I have included a photo of Mother with Bernard and a few of their friends on her fourth birthday—April 12, 1917. They are all cute as can be. A few of them are waving American flags, and that is probably in support of America's entry into World War I which took place six days earlier. Americans were so naive and buoyant at that time about the United States going to Europe and winning that war quickly. From Bicknell, Indiana, the family moved to Washington, Indiana, and that was probably in the early 1920s.

The year after I returned to Indianapolis, I wrote to Uncle Bernard in Florida and asked him to write me with some of his childhood recollections. I wanted to get the family history before memories passed away. Also, I enclosed a copy of the 1917 photo taken at Mother's birthday party. In November, 1992, I received his reply. The content, context, and atmosphere relate to the issue at hand, so I'm including portions of the letter.

Uncle Bernard wrote, "Dear Heydon, I have thought about you many times since receiving your Sept. 28th letter. The pictures you sent brought many happy memories even though I didn't recognize some of my young playmates. James David and his sister, Mildred, were our closest friends at that time. We never had a fight over anything, as one of us would always give in. It's a wonderful memory. Merom, Indiana, was my birthplace. As I recall, I used to say I was born on the banks of the Wabash River. I think the house we lived in wasn't far away, and I was too young to recall anything exciting there. I do recall our moving to Bicknell, Indiana while I was 5 or 6 yrs. old. It was there where we lived next door to Mildred and James David for a while—then moved about a block away in our new house. My mother and father later moved to Washington, Indiana where my father ran the Reel-Blue Lumber Co. It was a new lumberyard and my dad was part-owner and manager. About that time I was taking violin lessons and later playing in a little four- or five-piece band. We had a job to play at the Liberty Theater. I don't recall that we ever received money for our services, but we did get free admission to the shows. Also, I think all five of us had girl friends that came to the theater on the nights that we played during the comedy part of the show. We would all leave after the comedy and go to Williams' Drug Store for an ice cream cone. We were so bashful that the girls would walk together ahead of us, and we would meet them at the drug store. It was also during that time that my mother and father got to thinking about moving to Bloomington so Bernice and I could get a college education. My father got a job with a larger lumber company, and it was there that we settled down, and I finished high school and went to Indiana University. I think Bernice did too for a while before she and your dad got married. I got my library degree and around that time I wrote to TVA to apply for a library job. At that time they were setting up a Technical Library for use by the many engineers and other technical people employed to work there. That was the best move I ever made because it was there that I met my future wife, Evelyn Maudlin, who had gotten a secretary job about the time I came there....Since this letter was started Nov. 15th it's time to sign off. Thanks again for your letter. – Bernard Foy"

Now, to supplement Uncle Bernard's memory, it was in 1929 the Foys moved from Washington, Indiana, to Bloomington, Indiana, the home of Indiana University. Robert was their third child, so they were now a family of five. The reason for the move to Bloomington was the concern for their kids' college education as Uncle Bernard wrote. Giving up their home and the lumber business in Washington was a sacrifice the parents were willing to make for their kids' education and future.

Once in Bloomington, Grandpa Foy bought a house and had some extra rooms which they rented to college students—a common practice at IU. Mother still had two years of high school left and finished them at Bloomington High School (B.H.S.). One of her classmates at B.H.S. and then at IU was Ross Lockridge, Jr., the author of the immensely popular mythic saga and 1948 literary sensation, *Raintree County*.[1] The book was hailed at the time by at least one critic as the Great American Novel. The atmosphere of the land, schools, and people I've mentioned above served as part of the backdrop for *Raintree County*, and that makes the story relevant here. It was a point in time but the essence continues in some degree to this day.

On June 26-27, 1981, my parents went down to Bloomington and Bloomington High School for the 50th reunion of the Bloomington High School graduating class of 1931. Ross had passed away, but his widow, Vernice, was able to come. She and Mother then shared good memories of those times many years before. In her scrapbook, Mother had saved the program from the B.H.S. commencement exercises of 1931, and it listed Ross as giving the class oration, entitled *The Tributaries*. Bernice also saved the program from the B.H.S. 1932 commencement which listed Vernice as a graduate that year.

I find *Raintree County* most appropriate to reference here, for it represented a vision of a world away from the world as we commonly know it. It's especially fitting that *Raintree County* was set in the Heart of the Heartland. Geographically and historically, the story is centered in a town northeast of Bloomington, but I find the atmosphere of Bloomington, where Ross and Vernice spent so many romantic and formative years, to be pervasive in the poetic rendering of the area's soul.

For those who aren't acquainted with Bloomington and the IU campus, I should mention that it is a most beautiful area. The rolling hills of southern Indiana; the deciduous forests with graceful leaves of many colors and shapes that hold residents, students, visitors, and artists in awe; the old limestone buildings of the university; the scholarly air, as well as the youthful student melee that permeate the campus. All of these have contributed to a very romantic and desirable lifestyle. A number of students never left the area after graduating from college. Bloomington can entice you, grab hold, and sometimes not let you go. There are world-class cultural offerings in this small city. The 1979 film *Breaking Away* is about life in the Bloomington area for IU students and the town locals. It was written by a former IU student—Steve Tesich—who had Bloomington deep in his blood. He won the Academy Award in 1980 for Best Writing, Screenplay Written Directly for the Screen.

Similar to countless thousands of other students who have gone to IU from the nineteenth century on, I know what it is to fall in love in Bloomington. It is truly intoxicating—living in a beautiful wonderland in a world of idealism. Things were a little tougher there during the Depression than during my time in the mid-1960s, but the exuberance and optimism of youth, as well as the beauty and atmosphere of the area, helped to buffer some financial hardships.

As an adolescent in Florida, I was perusing my father's library one day looking for something to read. Dad walked by, picked out *Raintree County* and handed it to me, saying, "Why don't you read this? It's about Indiana and written by someone we knew at IU. Mother was in his class at high school also." I did read the story and was amazed at the poetic beauty of it. I asked Mother more about Ross.

"Well," she said, "Ross and I were in the same class in high school and knew each other, but I was better friends with his girlfriend who later became his wife—Vernice Baker."

"How did your friendship start?"

"I believe that it was because our names were so similar. She was Vernice, and I was Bernice—only the first letter was different. Vernice was a year younger, so she was in the junior class while Ross and I were seniors."

"I remember that sometimes we would double-date. The boy I was dating had a car, so he and I would be in the front seat while Ross and Vernice would ride in the back. We would be driving along and then I would suddenly hear Ross reciting poetry to Vernice. It was very romantic. Ross was extremely smart. They were both very nice, and we always had a good time together." I believe that Ross and Vernice served as models for the hero and heroine of *Raintree County*. Mother couldn't have known that the poetry she heard recited would set the tone for an immensely popular and meaningful novel.

It was in this atmosphere and period that my parents met, fell in love and committed themselves to one another. Their meeting happened like this. Mother's parents rented some rooms to students as I mentioned earlier. One of those students was a good friend of Dad's. He started telling my father of the nice, pretty young lady who lived where he rented a room. Finally, Dad went home with his friend one day when Bernice was going to be there. They met, and that was that. Mother's scrapbook documented their courtship.

Bernice saved a program from a musical play "The Only Girl" put on by "The Dramatic Board of Control of Indiana University" at Assembly Hall on March 29-30, 1933. At the bottom of the program she wrote, "Buck took me…started to date him Feb. 25, 1933—Tea Dance in Union Building." They were both nineteen years old then—perfect age and perfect locale to fall in love. Funny enough, the same thing happened to me when I was nineteen and attending IU Bloomington.

Two days before their date to the play, Mother had another experience which was probably more exciting but also very threatening. She and two of her friends were held hostage during a holdup at the Indiana Theater in Bloomington. I never imagined Mother in a situation like that until I saw her scrapbook after she passed away. She never spoke about it to me. This gentle soul just took the incident in stride. Mother had saved two newspaper articles about the holdup published the next day, Monday, March 28, 1933. In Bloomington this incident was a very big deal. Both newspapers had front-page, bold headlines spread across the top of the page. One paper wrote: "GUNMEN GET $500 AT INDIANA THEATER." The other read: "4 BANDITS GET $500 AT INDIANA THEATER."

The essence of the story was that Bernice was sitting in the lobby of the new theater on Sunday, March 27th, at 9:30 PM with two good friends—Thelma and Joe. Thelma's parents owned the theater. Two of the bandits—nicely dressed and unmasked—walked in. According to one newspaper, one of the bandits "walked up to Walter Bidwell, ticket taker, and pulling back Bidwell's coat, shoved a gun in his ribs and said quietly, 'This is a holdup. Walk on and don't make a false move.'"

Then he escorted Walter up the stairs to the office while another bandit stopped in front of Mother, Thelma and Joe, and "pulling his revolver ordered them up the steps behind Bidwell."

"Crouch [Joe] headed the line, Miss Foy was second and Miss Vonderschmidt [Thelma] third. About halfway up the stairs Miss Foy caught her heel and jerked her slipper off. When she fell slightly backward she pushed Miss Vonderschmidt back against the robber, who stuck his revolver against her back. Neither girl made an outcry and the robber picked up the shoe, assisted Miss Foy to put it on and remarked, 'This would be a joke in China.'"

That was a strange comment for a bandit to make. I assume he was speaking about the size 8 shoe since Chinese women often bound their feet—a painful process to keep the feet small.

"The outside office room was dark and the holdup men forced the little procession of prisoners into the inner office in which Mrs. Hays was standing."

"The tall man, who seemed to be the leader, said to her, 'Be quiet, it's just a little holdup.'"

"Scooping up all the cash in the office, the robbers walked out with the warning, 'Don't come outside this office for several minutes or you'll get plugged.'"

When I read this article, I thought it sounded like the language and actions of the 1930's gangster films we used to see—"Don't make a false move." "Don't come outside this office for several minutes or you'll get plugged." So I guess people really spoke that way, especially in

1933. Of course this was the time period of John Dillinger, and he robbed banks in this general area.

The newspaper article concluded, "The group who witnessed the holdup were not harmed by the episode with the exception of Miss Vonderschmidt, who has been very nervous since an automobile accident a few months ago in which she received a severe concussion of the brain. The shock of the robbery made her very nervous, and she was unable to attend school today." So Mother and Joe went on to classes as usual the next day, and the following day Mother and Dad went to the play. Sounds like my gentle, soft-spoken mother just took it all in stride.

Less than two weeks later, Bernice got a note from the Dean saying that she had a "D" at mid-term in history and that she should confer with her teacher. I think the grade is pretty understandable with all that happened in her life in the previous month. At the bottom of the Dean's note, Mother wrote, "Final grade was a C."

So going out with a bang and not a whimper, Bernice Foy finished that semester, completed her two-year college teaching certificate, and moved to Franklin, Indiana to begin teaching. Dad was on a four-year program and had one year left at Bloomington, having skipped a grade in school and starting college the month after he turned seventeen. After graduation, Buck got a job with General Electric. He and Bernice married in March, 1938, in a little church which was close to campus and had meant so much to them.

Their first child, Edith Ann, arrived eighteen months later. Then the rumbles of war began, and Buck was drafted. Following his ROTC training at IU, he had become a commissioned reserve officer and now began his service as a young infantry officer. He was inducted at Fort Benjamin Harrison in Indianapolis. During WWII, Mother and Edith Ann lived with her folks who had moved to South Bend, Indiana.

Dad went first to England and Ireland for some training before going on to North Africa and the combat push across the continent, then Sicily, and all the way up Italy. He was overseas over thirty-six months before receiving a leave near the end of the war. During his time overseas, he and Mother wrote each other most every day. I have a large number of V-mails and letters from those days. It is very touching to read of these young loves being separated and thinking of each other.

He also wrote so much in query about "the baby." Ann was certainly a much-loved child and another strong impetus for Buck to return alive.

In May of 1945, the European portion of WWII ended, and Dad returned to the United States. He had truly excelled as a soldier and went from second lieutenant to lieutenant colonel, moving from the field to G-2 intelligence and working on General Mark Clark's Command Staff. He also served as a liaison with 15th Army Group headed by Field Marshal Harold Alexander—a soldier's soldier as described by Buck; probably a father figure for Dad whose own father had died when Dad was fifteen.

Returning to the U.S., Buck decided to stay in the army and was assigned to the Pentagon. He and Mother rented a home in Bethesda, Maryland before buying a house in Washington, D.C. In a conversation in later years he told me that the money he used for a down payment on that house was money he had won at poker overseas. He didn't say that he was particularly good at poker, but that he was lucky.

A year after he returned to the U.S., Dad was on top of the world: the war was over; he had survived and come back as a conquering hero; he was a rising star at the Pentagon with a blossoming career; he was back with his beloved wife and daughter; and now he had a new child—me. Life was good.

The next step in his career was another plus. He was assigned to teach at the prestigious Command Staff and War College at Ft. Leavenworth, Kansas. As he described that period in later years, I could tell that he was very proud of that assignment. It meant that one was highly recognized and respected by peers and superiors. The plaque awarded to instructors there was especially handsome—a mahogany shield with an engraved copper plate mounted on it.

A second award that meant a lot to him was his Member of the British Empire (M.B.E.) Award. That one came with a proclamation signed by the King of England. Buck was modest about the medals he had won, but this one was something special to him. With a half smile, he said to me, "They didn't hand these out to everyone." The M.B.E. was awarded for his role in planning the invasion of Sicily since he worked very closely with British Command and had been lauded by them.

*****

From the Command Staff and War College, the family went on to the Army Language School (now called Defense Language Institute West Coast—DLIWC) at Monterey, California. He was assigned to a Russian language class, and we rented a house in Carmel. He got a kick out of talking about Carmel in the late 1940s with the celebrities out walking to the post office to pick up mail or cruise around. The houses had no street numbers but only names—house name or family name.

Finishing language school, he packed up the family, and we headed back to Washington where he took another advanced intelligence course. Then he was assigned to the Pentagon war room with his area of specialty as Soviet Affairs. Mother gave birth to a set of twin girls soon after arriving in Washington, so now Buck and Bernice had four children.

The cold war began, and intense political pressure was about to affect Buck's life—and that of his family—forever. Mother's role as the stabilizing element in the family was about to come into play. This was the time period of Senator Joe McCarthy and his campaign against Communism—his witch hunt with nonsense claims that many army officers and State Department personnel were card-carrying Communists. The hostilities had begun in Korea; the Red Scare had begun in Washington; and a ruthless politician was holding court.

As a reference to the severity of the pressure in Washington that he and others faced, Dad would mention the case of Secretary of Defense James Forrestall. The Secretary suffered a nervous breakdown from the pressure. Taken to Walter Reed Army Hospital for recuperation, Secretary Forrestall found an unlocked window one night in the snack room on the sixth floor. When no one was around, he jumped out of that window to his death. The whole situation must have been intense as we've seen somewhat in movies depicting the era, but Army and State Department employees in Washington were really in the worst of the cauldron.

The Korean War went into full gear a little later, and Buck was given his orders to Korea. In terms of pressure, it turned out that he was going from the frying pan into the fire. After a term of duty in the field, he was rotated back to Koje-Do Prisoner of War (POW) Camp as the commanding officer of security for the camp. He commanded the military police battalion, as well as the South Korean guards who were also stationed there to guard the North Korean and Chinese POWs. The prisoner population had rapidly expanded to 170,000 POWs; yet there weren't proper facilities to house a fraction of that number.

Inadequate compound facilities and open, severe hostilities between guards and prisoners led to very bloody eruptions. The South Korean guards and North Korean POWs hated each other, and the guards would look for any excuse to shoot prisoners. Different factions within the prisoner compounds were at war and executions took place often. I heard that on some mornings the sewage troughs leading out from the compound were literally running red with blood. To say the least, it was a very bad nightmare for everyone.

While negotiators at Panmunjon were working on a resolution to the war, Buck was trying to keep the Koje mayhem in check, and it seemed a virtually impossible task. To the man who believed he could solve any problem, the immense pressure of keeping these various groups from killing each other was taking him to the edge of his ability and beyond. In the end, he did a pretty good job and was recognized by General Dodd for his actions. (I have a copy of the commendation letter.) However, Buck was never the same after. Nine days after Dad finished his tour of duty in Korea and rotated back to the U.S., General Dodd was captured by the POWs, and then the POWs had an audience on the world stage. It's quite an historical story.

On the one hand, this narrative of Buck's war experiences may not seem relevant to Mother and Alzheimer's disease. However, when a spouse becomes neurologically impaired—for example, through severe combat experience—the other parent has to assume more of the parental responsibilities and subsequently handle more pressure. In the case of our family, Mother had to draw even more on her own serenity to become a force of emotional stability in our upbringing. She did this quite well, and this is important to note in her development as a person, as well as a Mother. She also did this without sacrificing her laughter and joy and childlike enthusiasm for whatever adventures we were all involved in.

*****

When Buck returned from Korea, he retired from the army. Enough was enough. Personally, I believe that soldiers—even excellent, dedicated soldiers—may only have one war in them, especially if they've established a family between wars and settled into a non-combat life. When the black-and-white reasons and objectives for one war are followed by a mass of gray motives and objectives trying to justify a later undeclared war, a soldier's inner voice becomes even more persistent in asking, "What am I doing here?"

Dad joined us in Tampa, Florida, where Mother had brought their four children the year before. They bought a nice little house in an old, established neighborhood with a bunch of friendly neighbors. Tampa, in the early 1950s, was a sleepy little city—a semi-tropical port of balmy weather and gentle winds rustling the palm trees and warming the skin. After dinner, the adults from half dozen or more homes would take their folding chairs to one neighbor's yard and talk about the day and life. It was therapeutic for them, and they all bonded well. We kids would play games, run, and ride our bikes until darkness came. All of this was done in the long twilight dusk while the air was permeated with night-blooming jasmine.

For Dad, it must have truly been paradise. He had just come from the world of combat and the infamous, brutally-cold Korean winter where soldiers huddled together to stay alive. In later years, he told me of seeing soldiers break down because of the endless cold with some soldiers collapsing in the snow and crying. Also, a buddy system meant you kept an eye on your buddy's face to make sure frostbite hadn't started; nevertheless, frostbite caused the amputation of many limbs in Korea. The army, combat, POW nightmares, and killing cold were all behind him now; or at least far enough away from immediate thoughts to allow some recuperation. He got a job as editor of the Telephone Company's magazine *Hello* in downtown Tampa and happily took the bus to work daily so that Mother had the car for kids and errands.

One evening a few years later, when I was eleven, he took Mother and my sisters to a new movie—the musical *Porgy and Bess*. When they got home from the theater, he said, "Heydon, you should really see that film. It's so moving! So much heart!" Then he started singing one of the songs from the movie. He had a good voice, and he loved to sing, whether he was in the church choir or simply walking down the street. "Summertime, and the livin' is easy. Fish are jumping, and the cotton is high. Your daddy's rich, and your momma's good looking. So, hush little baby, don't you cry...." The power of the movie and music was a healthy dose of healing balm for him, and every little bit helped.

We kids were fortunate to have a nice roof over our heads, good food, loving parents, and a country free of war. Little wonder that our parents had us say our prayers at night. Sometimes I saw Dad as being like an often-rumbling volcano—subdued on the surface but building pressure steadily until something would set him off. It was periodic and unavoidable. Our salvation, especially at that point, was Mother's gentle strength and stability. She gave us a solid foundation during those times when it seemed that the world was falling apart.

*****

It would not further the purpose of this writing to detail more of our lives during the six years we lived in Tampa, the subsequent six years in Lakeland, and then the move back to Indiana. At some point in Tampa, Dad became known to friends more often as Bud than Buck; perhaps it was a softer feel for civilian life.

Our father had a heavy sense of responsibility, rarely missed work, and made sure we had a comfortable home. At the same time, he was always carrying the wounds of war. During our life in Tampa, he went to the VA for counseling and was diagnosed as having bipolar illness, called manic depression at that time. Whatever medications were available for that in the 1950s were relatively primitive and in any event they didn't work for him.

His friends, neighbors, and the community had little idea of his condition. He was a handsome, dashing figure who gave freely of his time and abilities to make a better community and a better world. He was a very complicated man who had a great head and heart, but he was seriously conflicted inside and remained so in one degree or another until the day he died.

When I saw the television news in 1973 showing the American POWs being released from Hanoi, I was happy for them and also for their families knowing that their husband/father/son would soon be

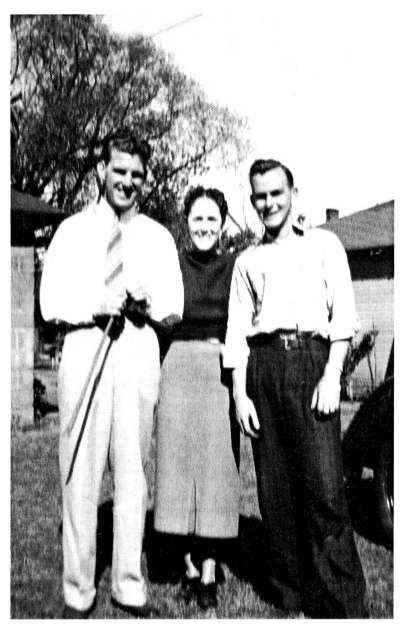

Buck and Bernice (two months married) with Bernice's
brother Robert on right. May, 1938, Mishawaka, Indiana

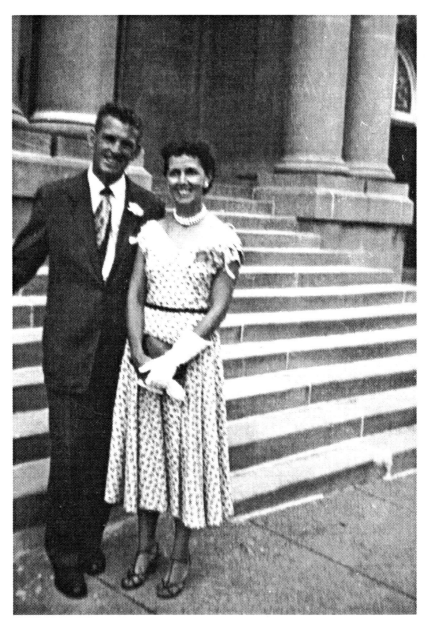

Buck and Bernice, circa 1939, Washington, Indiana
(at her cousin's wedding)

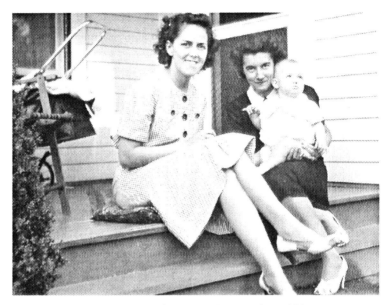

Bernice, Evelyn Foy (Bernard's wife)
and baby, 1940

Four generations—Bessie Foy, Grandma Pet, Bernice, and
Ann in front, 1944, South Bend, Indiana

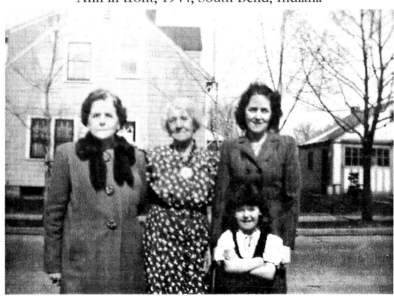

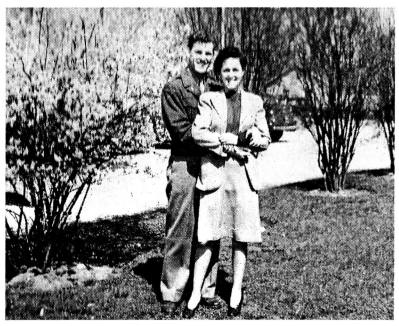

Buck and Bernice, early 1945, South Bend, Indiana
(Buck on leave from WWII—Italy)

Below: Buck, Ann, and Bernice

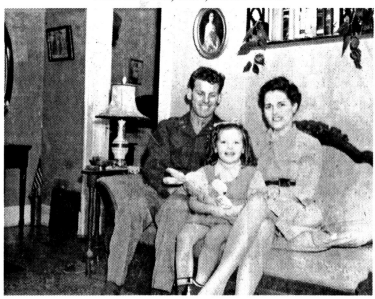

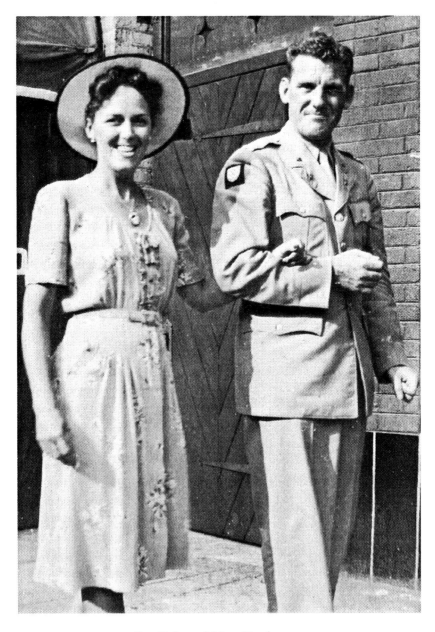

Lt. Col. and Mrs. Buchanan
August 12, 1945, Chicago, Illinois
(Young marrieds rejoined. WWII in Europe was over.)

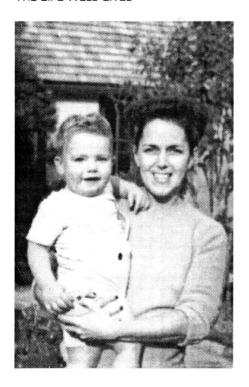

Heydon & Mother,
1948, Carmel, California
(Our home was in
Carmel while Buck
attended Army
Language School in
nearby Monterey to
learn Russian.)

Bernice, circa 1950,
Washington, D.C.

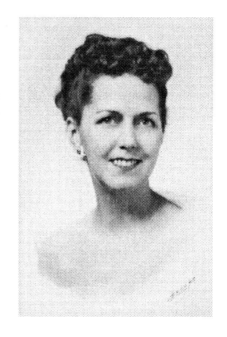

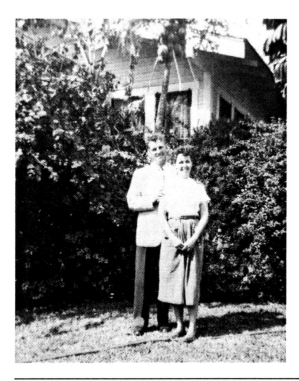

Buck and
Bernice,
circa 1954,
home in
Tampa, Florida

Back from
Korea,
in from
the cold,
retired from
the army.

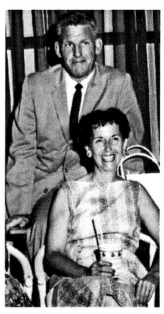

Bud (Buck) and
Bernice, 1962,
Daytona Beach,
Florida

(Vacation trip
while living in
Lakeland, Florida.)

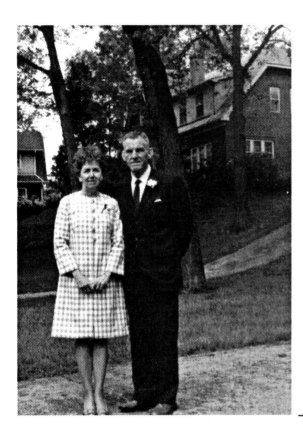

Bernice and Bud,
circa 1966,
home on
Watson Road,
Indianapolis,
Indiana

Left: Bud; Right: Bernice; Center: foreign graduate
student they sponsored through their church. 1967

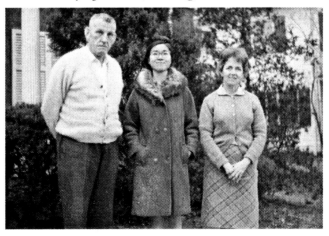

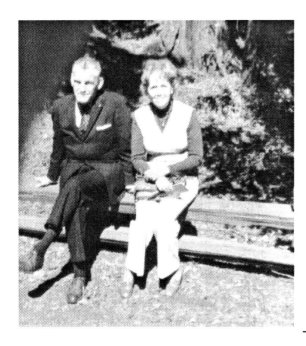

Bud and Bernice,
1973,
Muir Woods,
California

Bernice and Bud, February, 1978,
The trailering adventures—various trips from the Heartland:
northeast to Nova Scotia; south to Florida;
southwest to Arizona; west to the Rose Bowl;
and then through Mexico on a caravan.

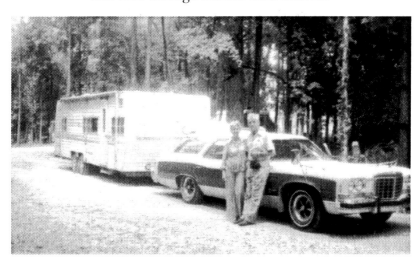

Back home again
in Indiana,
October, 1977.
Soon, the snow-
birds will trailer
off for the winter.

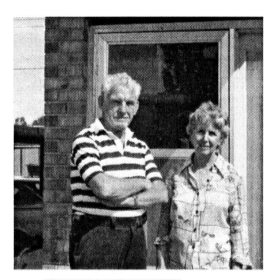

1979,
Indianapolis.

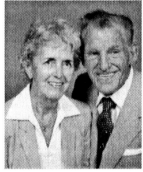

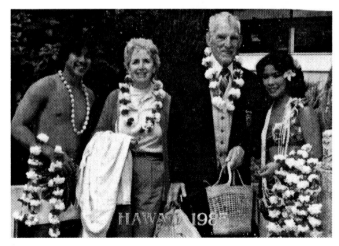

Bernice
and Bud
off to
visit
Hawaii,
1985.

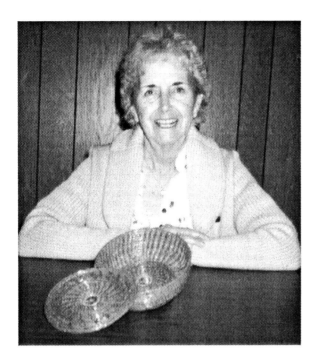

1983 Winter, Florida, Learning to weave pine needle baskets, adding to her many craft skills.

Bernice, Bud, and daughter Ann, late 1980s.
So many years they had shared together.

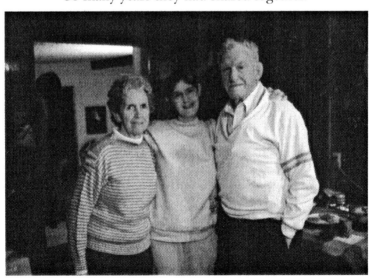

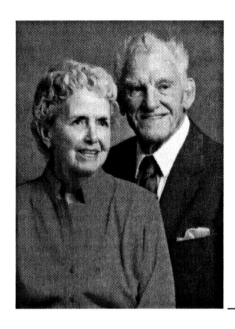

March 2, 1988
50th Wedding Anniversary.
Vows retaken at
Ft. Benjamin
Harrison Chapel

Celebration below was at Fort Harrison Officer's Club.

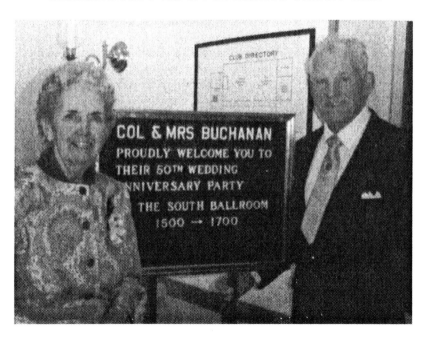

home. At the same time, I was concerned about what those families may have ahead of them in terms of readjustment—for the former POWs as well as their wives and children. The price of war goes well beyond the costs of military training, equipment, munitions, soldier deaths and physical disabilities, civilian deaths, and the anguish of families on the home front. The lingering plague involves the mental and emotional wounds that come home with the soldier. In World War I it was called shell shock; in World War II and Korea it was termed combat stress or battle fatigue; and after Vietnam it was coined post traumatic stress disorder (PTSD). My father was a victim of PTSD or battle fatigue.

*****

Spouses and children of the returning "walking wounded" heroes are often confused when these soldiers suddenly blow up in the home environment. Further, the families have often blamed themselves for the anger and insanity they witness, feeling that someone so highly regarded by society could not be at fault. Children often assume the blame for a parent's visible problems or discontent. You can try to convince them otherwise, but it's difficult. My sisters and I were fortunate to have our mother as a stable force to help us through those times, to at least try and tell us that it wasn't our fault. She never showed anything less than full love and respect for Dad and expected us to do the same. I don't think Dad could or would appreciate Mother's efforts at those times because in the midst of his emotional chaos, he didn't like himself at all. It wasn't any easier for Mother to understand his troubled behavior than it was for us. However, she tried to always do it—to follow her marriage vows and to help the man she loved. At the same time, she worked just as hard to protect and love us kids. She had her hands full. It was very fortunate for Dad and us that Mother's character was serene by nature. From my earliest recollection until the day she died, she continued on this path of love and compassion that helped all of us survive and often find happiness together.

Both of my parents were heroic. My father's achievements were more obvious to the public eye and subsequently received more praise. He didn't consciously brag of his accomplishments, but he did enjoy the attention when it came his way. My mother's sacrifices were more subtle and out of public view, and I don't believe she even considered them sacrifices. She saw them as doing the right thing, and this was reward in itself. She found happiness in that and didn't rely on reinforcement. I don't believe any of her children have reached that level.

To my knowledge, Bernice hadn't read Dr. Schweitzer's comment, "Living by example is not the main thing in influencing others, it is the only thing." Mother already knew this in her head and heart. It was inherent with her, and worked from the inside out.

*****

The life of Bernice Buchanan is a study of a person who lived a self-sacrificing life, giving endlessly, selflessly, joyfully. She knew the secret to life—the value of love. She found her work; she did it lovingly and without expectation of recognition. I believe she lived on a higher plane than most of us, and that was manifested in her demeanor and contributions to the world. She lived her faith but never spoke of it. Many of us seek gurus or mystics as teachers because they have supposedly risen to a much higher spiritual level. Some of those idols may be spiritually advanced, others may not be. However, the point is that we have access to teachers in our daily lives, but we don't usually slow down enough to recognize them or the lessons they offer by example.

The true jewels in our society are not found in the world of celebrities and other media faces that are fed to the masses. The real gems are those individuals who live in inner harmony and serve the world silently without need or desire for recognition. They know who they are as people, as members of the human race, and as children of God. Bernice Ione Foy Buchanan was one of those gems.

Knowing Bernice made life worth living. She gave her life in service for our family and for many other people as well. Now it was time for me to repay her to the best of my ability.

CHAPTER 4

ARRIVING—
HOME IS WHERE THE HEARTS ARE
(1991-1995)

A man travels the world in search of what he needs and
returns home to find it.
   —George Moore

Wherever a man may happen to turn, whatever a man may
undertake, he will always end up by returning to that path
which nature has marked out for him.
   —Unknown

IN EARLY MARCH 1991, I CROSSED THE STATE LINE FROM ILLINOIS
into Indiana. I was just a few hours from Indianapolis and home.
Back home again in Indiana... so goes the classic Hoosier song—the one
that is sung by Jim Nabors at the beginning of the Indianapolis 500 each
year. Much more than just the preface to the green flag on race day, the
song says something of life in the Hoosier state as well or perhaps the
life of yesteryear here.

The song has a universal application as well. While researching, I
learned that singers have covered it from Rosemary Clooney to Bobby
Darin to Neil Diamond to Louis Armstrong to the Grateful Dead and
beyond; now that is some variety, and the list doesn't even include the
instrumentalists who have covered it. Why is there such a lure? My guess
is that it is a call to return home, to come back to a mythical place and
era where things were pure and simple. Indiana was a perfect setting for

it. The song was written by James Hanley in 1917. The complete lyrics are as follows:

Back home again in Indiana,
And it seems that I can see
The gleaming candlelight, still shining bright
Through the sycamores, for me.

The new mown hay sends all its fragrance
From the fields I used to roam;
When I dream about the moonlight on the Wabash,
Then I long for my Indiana home.

My father would just start singing this at times, always with a smile. Maybe he would hear someone else start it, or he'd be watching IU basketball, or other references to Hoosier life could bring it on. It was always nice to see him with happy, uninhibited singing. As a kid I would be embarrassed when we were walking along the street, and he'd start singing heartily. I learned to accept it. Now I find myself singing that way, and my wife, when walking with me, is in the role I used to fill—the role of being at least slightly embarrassed.

What an interesting brew of people have come from the state of Indiana—Cole Porter and Hoagy Carmichael, Ernie Pyle and Booth Tarkington, James Dean and Red Skelton, Jim Jones and Charles Manson, Ross Lockridge, Jr. and Gene Stratton Porter, Theodore Dreiser and Kurt Vonnegut, Larry Bird and John Mellencamp, John Dillinger and William Henry Harrison, Wes Montgomery and James Whitcomb Riley, Madame Walker and Dan Wakefield, Eugene V. Debs and the John Birch Society, Andy Jacobs, Jr. and Dick Lugar, Tippicanoe and Tyler too, and on and on and on…not to mention Bud and Bernice Buchanan.

There's something about the fertile soil, the weather, and the heart in this area that nourish some basic, good values. There's also an undercurrent of individualism and rebellion which can produce famous people of extremes as listed above. Perhaps the most notable human contribution from Indiana was Abraham Lincoln. At least he spent his most formative years in the state—ages seven through twenty-one. One quote from Abe in recognition of the principal character in this book: "All that I am, and all that I may become, I owe to my angel mother."

He was truly a great man. For those of us on a much lower level of achievement, and without Mr. Lincoln's unique character and abilities, we still recognize the importance that mothers have played in our lives, and the honor they deserve.

The line in the "Indiana song"—*When I dream about the moonlight on the Wabash*—speaks of an earlier, more peaceful, and innocent age in the state's [and country's] history—a time and place that so aptly describes Bernice. She was born in Merom in the early part of the twentieth century at the highest Indiana point overlooking the Wabash River, four years before the song was written in 1917. The songwriter was probably looking down from Merom Bluffs, that best of vantage points for seeing "moonlight on the Wabash."

Another example of Hoosier writing during the early twentieth century was by the well-known poet James Whitcomb Riley. His poems—for example, "Little Orphan Annie" and "Barefoot Boy"—also represent the tenor of the time in Heartland Americana.

When I was a youngster, and bored one day while looking for something to do, I asked Mother what she did for fun in her early years. She suddenly looked beyond me and into the distance, then smiled and said in a hushed, but emphatic voice, "Chautauqua! We had Chautauqua."

Her reply really caught my attention—what she said and how she said it. Suddenly I was transported from my bored-child condition into her excited recall of that mythical yesteryear. My first thought was, "Wow! My mother speaks an Indian language." Just from her pronunciation of that one word—"Chautauqua!"—and the style of her reply, I was assuming that she could be fluent in the language. She spoke it just like a native—an American Indian. When I heard her reply, I was suddenly transported back to the American Indians of the eighteenth-century northeastern United States and *The Last of the Mohicans*. Now drawn in, I had to learn more about "Chautauqua!" It turned out to be another institution from yesteryear. Chautauqua was like a traveling cultural center for rural America—forums for popular education combined with entertainment in the form of lectures, concerts, plays, art classes, children's activities, and on.

As I understand it, Chautauqua was first implemented in upstate New York around 1875. It was designed to serve as a process of renewal—for family life, mind and spirit, intellectual curiosity and social interaction, and freedom of individual religious expression. There were also political speakers, as well as inspirational speakers—people who had met and mastered great adversity. All this was done in a natural and healthy atmosphere away from town and city. People could tent or rent rooms or cottages. There were hundreds of Chautauquas in the country, and they might stay in an individual area for two weeks before moving on. One of the biggest was the Merom Chautauqua, and that was the one Bernice's family attended.

Some of the speakers were Billy Sunday, William Jennings Bryan, Helen Keller, Eugene V. Debs, Warren Harding, and Carrie Nation. Another was Booker T. Washington who told of his rise from slavery. How incredible it must have been to listen to a speech written and delivered by Booker T. Washington! Or Helen Keller! Or Eugene Debs!

A number of inspirational books were written about Chautauqua. One writer, Isabella Alden, wrote a few of them—*Four Girls at Chautauqua*, *The Chautauqua Girls at Home*, and *Four Mothers at Chautauqua*. It was a time of wholesome innocence in rural America, and these events would have been especially romantic to young girls who could meet boys from other towns. In summary, President Theodore Roosevelt called Chautauqua "the most American thing in America." Chautauquas began to die out in the early 1900s as the Hollywood film industry offered the new entertainment. Another contribution to their demise was the advent of the automobile, which gave people the freedom to easily travel long distances, at their convenience, to other entertainment.

*****

Arriving in Indy, and then the parking lot of Mother's townhouse, I turned off my truck and thought how different it would be to enter and not find Dad there. I had called Mother when I crossed into Indiana, and she said she'd be at home and didn't plan to go anywhere. She came to the door after my knock and had a big smile on her face. "Well," she said, "I thought it was you." We hugged, and I went in to sit and have a cup of coffee while we spoke about the trip.

"I'm very happy to have you here," she said. It's nice to have a welcome reception like that.

"I'm very happy to be here," I replied.

There was never any question in my mind about how we would get along. We were of the same temperament and enjoyed each other's company. If we had been very different, I probably wouldn't have moved back for the caregiving.

I called a few people to let them know I had arrived, and said that I was at Mother's home. After the second call and hearing me say, "I'm at Mother's home," Mother said, "You know this is your home, too." She really wanted to make a point of that.

"Thank you," I replied. She was so sincere and wanted me to be very comfortable.

Later I took my luggage into the extra room upstairs where I would be sleeping. It had been a study for Dad. His library was still there, as well as various wall hangings—photos of army times, the family, and other frameables he had collected along the way. His desk was there and also an old pullout sofa. When I did open the sofa to make a bed, there was very little space left to walk around it. That would be fine, as it was just a room to sleep.

During the next few days, I settled in and tried to gauge the extent of Mother's memory problem. She assured me everything was fine, and that she didn't have much of a problem. She would repeat some things within the course of a few hours, sometimes adding, "I may have told you that already." Again, we were both of similar temperament so I knew intuitively not to say "You already said that," or "You just asked me that question," or some other inconsiderate response. Aside from the point of compassion, I also wouldn't be able to gauge her problem very well if I inhibited her with some reproach that reminded her of the forgetfulness. Even after her diagnosis and more time passed, I never brought up the repetition when she asked me the same question several times in a row. I just simply answered the question as though it was the first time she had asked it, and finally she would stop asking.

I had some ideas or theories that I wanted to try first before considering the possibility of an irreversible and progressive dementia. This was not denial of a serious dementia problem because there simply had not been a diagnosis when I arrived. There were other things going on. Her mate of fifty-three years had died less than two months earlier. She assured me she was feeling okay on that point. My father had many good qualities, but he was also an often driving and impatient man, at least toward his immediate family—his wife and children who were the people most around him, and whom he loved most. He was even harder on himself, but that was of no relief to us.

My theory on Mother's condition was that without his pressure on her, she would relax more easily, and subsequently her short-term memory might improve. Of course, I should add that his impatience rarely threw her visibly off-balance; so my assumption was based on the idea that his continued needs might have affected her internally without changing her outward demeanor. This was an idea I had considered during the drive from L.A. So, my plan was to create as tranquil and easygoing an atmosphere as possible in the townhouse. With Mother and me, this would happen automatically.

However, if a sibling of mine was having a turbulent marital relationship, I didn't want that turbulence transferred to Mother's home. Mother didn't need to be a repository for other people's perennial woes. It's one thing to have a problem and discuss it reasonably; it's another matter to carry and demonstrate one's anger in another person's home; that is simply transference—an immature action at best. Some may consider my actions as being overprotective, but I didn't want Mother—this most gentle soul—to be burdened with someone else's anger, especially when a stable atmosphere was needed to determine the degree of Bernice's memory loss.

I had taken the tranquility idea a step further. I was going to make a professional sign to hang over the front door to read "Casa de Paz"—House of Peace. I pursued the peace idea not because I expected problems but simply as a preventive measure should they happen to reach the front door.

There was really only one incident of a somewhat heated nature during my years there. One of my sisters was preaching to Mother one day, a bit of fire and brimstone. Mother was patient, nodded her head in acknowledgment, and gave an occasional "Um," or "Uh huh."

I couldn't stay quiet and began to question my sister's points, and we started getting a bit argumentative. Anyone who believes that their particular dogma is the only path to the kingdom of God is off-track to my thinking.

After my sister left, Mother said to me, "Heydon, I don't understand why you do that."

"Do what?" I asked.

"Argue with her like that. Why can't you just let it be?"

"Well," I replied, "she thinks her religion is the only way to God, and it bothers me."

"She's just talking," Mother replied. "It doesn't hurt anything. Let her talk." My parents had always advocated freedom of religion and allowing their children to express themselves.

"Okay," I answered, "you're probably right." And Mother was right. I thought Mother was being exploited as a captive audience for the sermon, but in fact Mother was just giving her daughter the chance to express herself as she wanted. Mother was wise while I was reactive. Some childhood dynamic may have also played into my reaction. This is probably a case where I was overprotective, but I was also aware of Mother's gentle nature and increasing vulnerability.

I had gotten tired of hearing this sibling preaching over the years. I had reached my limit. I especially didn't want her sermonizing to Mother who was, without doubt, the truest example of Christianity I had ever seen or known. Watching her preach to Mother was like seeing a flamboyant, bejeweled televangelist lecturing down to Mother Teresa on the essence of Christianity. There's just something very wrong with that picture.

A couple of my sisters had told this sibling to keep her views to herself, so she didn't bother them. I should have done the same long ago. I don't believe everyone in her religion pushes his or her opinion to the extent this sibling did, so there may have been some family dynamic involved as well.

At first, this matter of dogmatic religion may not seem relevant to the issue at hand, but bear with me as it will take on much more relevance in the issue of family dynamics and caregiving as discussed in later chapters.

Caregiving Assistance and Resources

During that first week back in Indy, I took inventory of what I could do to help Mother—to make her life easier, not only with regard to the memory issue but just day-to-day living. She could be left alone at this point.

My practical benefits to her at that time were first to give her a sense of security from problems of the outside world; for example, her being viewed and targeted as an elderly widow living alone, an easy mark. Beyond that, I ran phone interference for her. The telemarketers and insurance salesmen must have gotten her widow status from public records or the newspaper and were calling quite often to sell one thing or another. Mother was so gentle and considerate that they kept her on the phone quite a while even when she did say no.

I did some of the shopping and cooking also. That gave her a break. I was a fair cook at that point. Concerning the shopping, I went with her to shop, or did it myself if she wanted. The point of all this was to help her as much as she liked without simply doing it for her. Growing old is difficult enough without someone also taking over your life. So I wanted to assist as much as possible without imposing. The same principle carried over to caregiving as the dementia got worse—to help her as much as possible without sacrificing her dignity.

She could still do some laundry, and that was good. It gave her a sense of accomplishment that we all need to feel productive. She had worked so hard, endlessly and joyfully, all her life so that was just part of who she was.

Now, concerning personal resources to carry out my caregiving, I did an inventory of what was needed, and what I had available. I'm a very private person and wouldn't normally mention some of the following information; however, if it can potentially help another person in his or her decision to become a family caregiver, then it's worth offering.

First and foremost to consider were financial resources; that is, what I brought with me and had at my disposal, as well as what work opportunities and subsequent income were available in Indianapolis. Financially, my means were moderate. I had my savings, two small investments, and my IRA. I was willing to spend whatever it took in order to fulfill my commitment to her welfare.

My truck was new, and I had paid it off before leaving California. With the truck, I purchased a five-year full warranty, so there wouldn't be any potential problem with repair bills for a long time. My auto insurance would cost half of what it did in California. That was a relief. And I reduced the policy to low mileage coverage since I wouldn't be driving that much.

In my final year in California, I had started a separate business—a small venture in postcards, greeting cards, theme booklets, and frameables. While I didn't have the capital to develop the business further, I still had produced some inventory that I could sell locally. Conveniently, there was a shop close by that would handle the products. That could produce a little additional income.

Concerning expenditures, there were some important things to consider. By leaving L.A., I had given up my medical and dental insurance. Those were important items. If disaster struck me on the health front, my financial assets would be very vulnerable. As for medical treatment, there was a VA hospital here. With my active duty time in the army, I was entitled to some treatment there. Actually, it meant going to the emergency room for any treatment, since a regular doctor couldn't be assigned unless a veteran had disability from service. This was to change at the VA a few years later, as they suddenly had to compete with other medical institutions for health care dollars, and they began luring veterans in for treatment. For the present, the VA emergency room was available to me with its four-hour wait. I was in excellent health, so I tried to avoid that VA experience unless absolutely necessary.

I was somewhat concerned with the loss of dental insurance. That was more my Achilles' heel in terms of health expenses. Within a couple of years I enrolled in a reduced fee dental service, but that had mixed results as I tried several different dentists. It cost me a couple molars. There's no point in drawing that out, as any potential caregiver will have to work that issue out for himself or herself.

There was no rent needed for my sleeping room. And, I would live very modestly overall. So, I figured my assets should carry me along. But the question I asked myself was, "For how long?" How long? That was the question. How long would this "process" last? In November 1991, eight months after my arrival in Indianapolis, Mother's neurologist diagnosed her with "dementia of the early-Alzheimer's type." At the time, I believe the expected lifespan after an Alzheimer's disease diagnosis was two to eight years. So, I assumed my work would take about five years. That lifespan range has since been extended considerably, and it lasted beyond that eight-year maximum in Mother's case.

The term "process" I used above seems detached and antiseptic. I suppose I didn't want to think in terms of how long until death, until my mother died. Even the thought of that loss would be too distracting from the task at hand. Frankly, I stayed so busy with the million-odd details of caregiving that I didn't think about death. Anyway, death would take care of itself; living and caregiving are the issues that would take serious time and work.

I've read that relatives of Alzheimer's patients are often in denial about their loved one having the disease. I don't believe that was a problem for me. I was fully committed to Mother's welfare, so the disease label was not that important; however, once the disease was formally diagnosed, we could more completely evaluate Mother's needs. With a diagnosis, a caregiver can develop a more guided strategy for the long run to help the patient and himself or herself.

The Tools of Caregiving

Beyond the inventory of medical and financial resources necessary for caregiving, it is most important to develop a strategy or set of tools to handle the task at hand. The day-to-day health tools for care recipient and caregiver have to be organized with flexibility, since matters can change quickly. For example, if the caregiver is injured or dies, what is the backup plan to provide for the care recipient?

The basic daily activities can include diet, exercise, medical care, and socialization. However, the most important force in helping someone through the tortuous maze of Alzheimer's disease is love; I will cover that more completely in chapter ten.

1. Diet. How could I uphold the caregiving commitment if I didn't stay healthy? During life in California, I had developed a pretty good health regimen for diet and exercise. I continued the general food style when I cooked at home so that Mother would have a balanced diet. She already ate fairly well, but her physical exam in late 1991 showed her cholesterol and triglycerides to be a little high; so, when I cooked for her I usually used chicken or fish instead of red meat. Also, I bought and cooked a variety of vegetables; and kept a mixture of fresh fruit on hand.

Bernice started every morning with bran cereal, and her digestive system stayed as normal and flowing as could be. When we were at the doctor's one time for her physical exam, her regularity was one of the questions he asked about. She was very bashful about answering and smiled slightly while saying, "Well, the morning bran works for me."

In 1992, I decided to start vegetable and fruit juicing for Mother and myself. That was a good method for getting maximum nutrition from fresh produce. The juices served as a supplement to her regular diet so that she still got plenty of fiber as well.

When I learned that the elderly have more trouble absorbing nutrients, I decided that high-nutrient juicing, a balanced diet, and a supplemental vitamin would be the best combination. To stay on track with her medical treatment, I told her doctor of my plan, and the dietary routine sounded okay to him.

About six months after I started juicing, I saw an ad in the newspaper that "The Juiceman"—Jay Kordich—would be at a local mall to do demonstrations on juicing. I went to see it and was sitting in the audience before the start of the show. He came down to the seating area, introduced himself to me, and asked if I would help him during the show, handing him the vegetables and fruits for his demos. Jay was a very nice, high-energy fellow, and it was a pleasure to work and talk with him. I learned some good nutritional tips also. A couple of weeks after the show, he had his organization send me a full set of his instructional cassette tapes as a thank you for my time and assistance.

There is one other change I added to her diet. After reading what the health pioneers had to say on the subject of water, I bought a one-gallon water distiller and made steam-distilled water with added trace minerals to have on hand. Sometimes Mother would use that water; sometimes she would just draw from the regular water faucet; but it was an improvement for her health regardless of how much she used.

2. Exercise. Exercise was another matter. For Mother, her principal exercise was our walking the perimeter of the townhouse complex after supper. We made other sporadic walks as well. She had had knee replacement surgery a few years earlier, so the walking was sufficient to aid her heart and not overburden her joints. She maintained a healthy weight, didn't smoke or drink, had normal blood pressure and pulse, and a great attitude.

I needed more exercise—for health in general, and also for the steadily increasing stress of caregiving. In California I had done high impact aerobics three or four times a week at night after work. Now, as though by Divine plan, there was a gym a stone's throw from Mother's townhouse so I could get a solid aerobic workout there. I mention Divine plan in the placement of the gym, but its development also took a great deal of work by Bill and Karen—the owners of the gym.

Step Aerobics was the single most important exercise for me. Light weight training was a helpful supplement also. Both were blessings in the therapeutic help provided. In Step, the combination of stimulating music, an energetic instructor, and a roomful of nice people made the workout a pleasure. The one-hour respite from caregiving was also helpful—relieving stress, balancing brain chemistry, burning some calories, staying fit, and subsequently making me a more effective caregiver. I recommend exercise and its value to everyone, but it can be invaluable to the Alzheimer's primary caregiver.

My Step classes were at the intense level, and most of the other participants were young ladies almost half my age—people who had stopped at the gym after work or school and were in need of a solid workout. I was always puzzled why more men wouldn't come to the class. It was high energy and suited me just fine.

Within a couple years, the stress of caregiving was overshadowed by the stress of sibling disagreement about caregiving. That will be covered in more detail in chapter five. The point is that the exercise became more important as the multiple stressors took a toll on me.

Some people would yell in Step class as things heated up, and our pulse rates rose. The instructors loved the outcries because it raised the energy level in the room. After a year or two, I started yelling myself and probably louder than the other participants. No one would have guessed the origin of my need to yell, for no one knew my situation; but my enthusiasm was appreciated, whatever the reason. What a perfect outlet I found—a place to yell, and be appreciated for it, as well as a healthy mode of relieving stress, balancing mind and emotions.

While I had dozens of Step instructors over the eleven caregiving years, there were two who were with me all the way through, and, they still are today. It would be hard to find two finer young ladies anywhere. Lynn and Alicia were starting college when they began teaching step at the gym, and that's when we met. Since that time, they both completed college; completed professional schools (physical therapy and law); got married; bought houses; had children; ran marathons; and on and on. They are close friends who spur each other to ever-higher accomplishments. They are both very friendly, strong, and have great attitudes. At their current rate of achievement, I would expect before long that Alicia will be mayor of the city, and Lynn will be in charge of the city's health care and/or fitness programs. I believe that Lynn and Alicia are part of that Divine plan I mentioned earlier; I'm grateful that we were all put on earth in the same place at the same time.

3. Socialization. Since the disease can easily lead to isolation for the care recipient and caregiver, it is important to maintain some social contact throughout the disease process. The care recipient should have social contact as long as he or she is comfortable with it. I mention that because at some point, or during transition to another stage, AD patients can be uncomfortable being around other people.

During the day, Mother continued her regular activities. She had so many of them: a weekly program at the Shepherd Center for seniors, often serving as a greeter; a sewing circle at her church; volunteering at the soup kitchen at her church; a monthly luncheon of the senior members of Tri-Kappa; garage sales with a friend or a daughter; sewing at home; babysitting for grandchildren; getting her hair done; shopping at the commissary; and on and on. She was still driving well, quite functional, and able to go about her business. She hid her increasing disability pretty well.

There were several fraternal organizations that Dad had belonged to, and they asked Mother to certain functions as the widow of a former member. She always wanted me to come along with her in these cases; I assume it made her more comfortable, and I already knew a number of the people in the organizations. Also, Dad was held in high esteem in those organizations, so Mother and I were both quite welcome.

Dad had been a Mason, and Mother was invited to attend a couple of dinners at his Masonic Lodge. So we went and enjoyed ourselves. The Retired Officers Association also asked us to a couple of their functions. Also, the National Sojourners Association asked us to brunch a couple of times. This organization is open to Master Masons who have served in the military as commissioned officers or senior noncommissioned officers.

Another organization inviting us to attend was the Masonic Home Kids. This was a more intimate and emotional group. Like Dad, other members of this group had lost their parents early in life, and, since their fathers were Masons, the kids were eligible to live at the Masonic Home in Franklin, Indiana. Dad and his three brothers went there to live in 1928 after the death of their father, since their sister was eighteen years old and able to live on her own. The Home Kids accepted Mother as one of their own since they had known her for much of their lives. The Home Kids Alumni Association is a tight-knit group of people who survived hard times without parents, and their emotional bonds and level of mutual trust are strong and heartfelt. They consider their entire membership of two hundred or so to be truly brothers and sisters. They are like members of a military combat unit who have survived a long campaign together. Mother and I enjoyed their annual gathering here in Indiana, and they were always interested in Mother's welfare, as well as appreciating that I was here for her.

Individual Friends

It is quite common for friends to drop—or minimize—contact with the care recipient and caregiver when Alzheimer's disease sets in. There can be various reasons given for this change, but I believe the bottom line is that such friendships were simply shallow. If friends can't stand by each other in difficult times, then what they really have is a relationship of convenience.

Concerning this caregiver, I had an uncommon experience. I have two exceptional friends here in Indianapolis, and their contact with Mother and me didn't disappear or even stay the same during my caregiving; they increased their contact and level of support. This support was not only in being available to listen to me when I felt exhausted, but also in spending time with Mother and treating her continuously with full dignity and affection.

Pat and I have known each other for forty-two years and have experienced a lot of life's wonders and woes together. Actually, our fathers met each other in 1930, so there's a solid familial connection in time and experience. Many people are amazed at the length and depth of our friendship. I met Nancy here in Indianapolis in 1993, two years after I had begun my caregiving commitment. She worked with my sister in medical research, and we met at the research center. We started seeing each other in May 1993, and were married in June 1997. Nancy and Mother got along great and were able to enjoy each other's company from the early phase of Alzheimer's disease on through the end. Both Pat and Nancy made a very positive difference in our lives throughout the long caregiving period.

One principal bond Nancy and I shared was that she was a caregiver as well. She worked full-time and went home to Greensburg on weekends to help her mother care for her father. Nancy's father was a stroke victim and bed-ridden.

Most of Mother's friends had passed away or retired to warmer climates. There were three living that I should mention. Her oldest friend, Gwen, was also a widow and lived about a hundred and fifty miles north of Indianapolis. She had Mother up to spend a couple weekends on her farm. Gwen, Marion, Bernice, and Buck had been students together at IU in Bloomington and knew each other from the early 1930s. They were good friends.

Mary. Shortly after my return to Indianapolis, Mother introduced me to her friend Mary. Mary was walking by the townhouse and stopped to say hello. She appeared to be a few years older than Mother. Mary was also a widow and lived alone two streets over in the same complex. Beyond that, she was also a member of the same service sorority as Mother, so they had gone together to the monthly luncheons of the Tri-Kappas.

Mary was tall and lean with an intense energy about her. Memory problems had begun earlier for her than Mother. I knew this from our occasional meetings—either when she would stop by to see Mother, or when we would meet Mary during our evening walks around the complex. When we first met, Mary was already beginning to get that look which says "I'm having a little trouble putting all this together." Episodes of fear, anger, and panic were not far away—results of the dementia and subsequent disability which were compounding faster by her living alone. Mother was concerned about Mary, as she was quite aware of Mary's increasing problems.

When we met Mary on the sidewalk, we would stop to say hello and chat for a moment. The most memorable of her chats actually happened on a couple of occasions due to her forgetting. I didn't mind, especially in this case. The talk went like this. With her increasingly worried look, Mary stared right into Mother's eyes and said, "Boy, you're lucky to have him here!" Mary couldn't remember my name since she was slipping fast. Mother would smile kind of sheepishly, looking down toward her feet, and say, "Yes, I know. I really am."

Needless to say, those comments made me feel much appreciated. They also reinforced the rightness of my decision in moving back, seeing that Mary's condition could soon be in store for Mother, too. While that short conversation might sound like a light exchange between friends, it really harbored an undercurrent of very strong emotions—fear from Mary and gratitude from Mother.

So, when that conversation was repeated again on another occasion, I happily sat back and listened. Recognition like this is very helpful to the caregiver, especially later in the disease when the stress levels climb drastically. At that point, any support or reinforcement is quite welcome, anything to help you stay on your feet and off the ropes or the mat.

Mary was relatively coherent then. As months passed and her disability progressed, she began to speak about people breaking into her home and living in the spare bedroom. She said they came in at night through the back door. Further, she said that they were taking things. (This matter of "taking things" is important in AD, and I'll elaborate on that later.) She asked if I would please come to her place and check the locks. I asked if the maintenance men had not checked them for her, and she said that the lock they put on hadn't stopped the intruders. Mother also asked me to check it since she could see how upset her friend was. So off we went to Mary's apartment.

The locks looked fine to me. The maintenance man had even added another lock to the sliding glass door. She assured me the intruders still got in, though she didn't understand how. Since the locks were okay, I asked how else these intruders could get in. She replied, "I don't know, they just do! They could be coming in through the walls. Please help me!" she begged. An exercise in futility, I thought, but I told her that I would go to the office and speak to the manager. At the office, they were well aware of Mary's concerns and her problems. They had been speaking with her daughter about Mary's condition, and now realized it was time to talk with the daughter again.

Not long after this, Mary was taken to a nursing home. She was unhappy with the nursing home, and a few months later her daughter transferred her to another facility. Mary was also unhappy there, but there she was to stay.

One day in early 1993, Mother drove up to visit Mary. Bernice was still driving then. Later she told me she had some trouble finding the place, but that was understandable in that the facility is tucked away through back road curves and a cul-de-sac. When Bernice returned home, she looked pale and shaken. She began to describe the place to me.

"I don't want to go to a place like that. Mary shares a room with someone else, and the beds are only separated by a sheet. You can hear everything." She could have added that it's just like a hospital bed without the service, and with a lot of old, infirm people in the hallways reaching out for help. Actually, that was an average, or better-than-average, nursing home; however, for someone who has created and lived in a warm, gracious, and loving home all her life, nursing homes are quite a serious shock. I knew she had been in nursing homes before; however, since AD had set in, the conditions were accentuated for her.

That was the only time I saw Mother show any fear about something in life. I believe it was not only the conditions of the nursing home, but what placement in a nursing home really meant to her—that a person was being abandoned to a facility to live out their life in a room without privacy and surrounded by a sea of moans, and then to finally die alone.

I restated to Mother that I would always be there to care for her. I wanted to offer that reassurance to ease whatever anxiety may be lingering in her after the recent nursing home experience. What I really wanted to tell her was that she would never end up in a nursing home. However, honestly, I couldn't say that. I would do all humanly possible to keep her out of the nursing home, but a one-caregiver battle against the throes of Alzheimer's disease seems bound to lose if the patient lives long enough.

Bernice came from a generation and environment where you took care of your elderly at home. This was a new world to her. Leaving a gracious home after a long, independent and productive life and then going to a nursing home must have been incomprehensible, not to mention heartbreaking. Going from a life full of love and being loved to a dismal atmosphere where so many people are often pitiably crying out for help is enough to shake a person quite a bit. Mary died a few months later. And she was alone.

Selma. Bernice still saw her old friend Selma occasionally. Both of them were fans of IU basketball. They were both tenured Hoosiers as well as IU alumnae. Neither of them got too excited during the ball games, but they enjoyed watching them. Mother invited Selma over to watch a few games, and I would make some dinner for them, usually soup and sandwiches to have while watching basketball.

Selma was sharp mentally and wasn't always very patient with someone who was slipping. Mother repeated a question a few minutes after asking it originally, and Selma then asked, "Bernice, don't you remember you just asked me that?" I'm sure she cared a great deal for Bernice, but at times she just wasn't very understanding. She probably saw Mother's future and just couldn't deal with it.

One night after the game and dinner, I walked Selma out to her car. She had a worried look on her face and spoke with serious concern.

"Heydon," she started, "what's going to happen to Bernice? What are you going to do?"

"I will take care of her here at home as long as possible," I replied. "When the caregiving is absolutely beyond my ability, I'll probably have to take her to a nursing home."

"Oh, no, Heydon, not your mother!" Selma answered. "She's such a lady!"

"I know," I replied, "but if she lives long enough, it will be beyond my ability to take care of her."

That reply from Selma was the first time I had heard real emotion in her voice in the thirty years I had known her. Selma studied people closely and spoke sparingly unless she knew them well. Even then, she expressed herself without much emotion, speaking in a measured monotone.

Suddenly I saw a new dimension to Selma. Formerly I thought of Selma and Mother's friendship as casual get-togethers. Now I heard for the first time of Selma's full respect for Mother. In her clipped style, Selma had expressed it best—"Your mother is such a lady." The combination of Bernice's character, demeanor, dress, personal habits, and the treatment of other human beings did in fact represent very much a lady. I then recollected that was what so many other people saw in her as well.

*****

It must be terribly fearful for the elderly to watch their friends being sent to nursing homes—not only the destination but also being of the age where they themselves are closer to that fate.

Two years before my father died, I was home on a visit. We were having breakfast and looking out the picture window next to the dining table. The view faced the nearby tennis court, and beyond the court was another row of apartments and townhouses. Dad pointed to an apartment in that area and said, "A few months ago, our neighbors over there left. A moving van pulled up to the door, loaded all the furniture for auction, and drove off. Then the couple came outside, got into a cab, and went to live in the nursing home. It was very sad to see."

Dad had a solemn look and tone of voice as he described this. He was visibly disturbed. Reality was setting in with him. Mother went about straightening up in the kitchen and didn't say anything. She wouldn't. She didn't like for him to dwell on death and disability, and especially during my vacation visits, especially since we'd covered the subjects so many times already. A few months after this conversation, I received the audio tape from Dad which I mentioned at the beginning of this book.

I'm sure Bernice did share his feelings about nursing homes, but she herself wouldn't ask me specifically to keep her out of one. Also, she wouldn't want Dad to ask that on her behalf. She simply didn't ask for things for herself.

Actually, Dad's wishes were second to my own in terms of taking care of Mother. Trying to arrange her care before his own death would help fulfill his own sense of responsibility. My decision to take care of Mother and keep her out of a nursing home as long as possible was entirely my decision. I had to answer to my daily conscience. Also, I wanted to act in a way that would make me comfortable reflecting on that choice when it came my turn to die.

4. Medication. Mother didn't take any medications. Her only medicine was bran flakes. She was the epitome of health in habits, appearance and attitude. Actually, she produced medicine for others in the love and joy she shared with all.

Concerning myself—the caregiver—I didn't take any medication when I began caregiving, nor for a while thereafter. Eventually, I did take a low-level anti-depressant for some time—when caregiving became very emotionally demanding, and it was augmented by even more stressful sibling conflict. I'm not sure how helpful the medicine was, but it seemed to lower the depression a bit. While I would have preferred to do without that medication, I also felt that it was acceptable as a tool in that phase of my commitment.

Many AD caregivers develop depression. For some, it can be very severe. The matter of taking, or not taking, an anti-depressant is an individual matter which each caregiver should review with his or her physician if and when caregiving and related issues become overwhelming. The absolute best anti-depressant I used was physical exercise. Diet, friends, and spiritual reinforcement were my secondary defense. Medication, when used, was the last tool in line.

From what I've read, some caregivers develop an unhealthy dependence on alcohol and tranquilizers. While each of those substances may have some therapeutic effect, it is easy to cross into the area of abusing them when caregiving stresses seem to mount exponentially. It's best to be open with your doctor about their use. Ultimately, if the caregiver is disabled, the care recipient is in real trouble.

The underlying force that made all of my caregiving possible was love, but I'm not sure if that fits in this area of medication. Love wasn't something I took or did for myself. It was something that emanated from within and directed my actions in caregiving. Love was also something that flowed from the care recipient to me in her appreciation for being helped.

5. Siblings? Some of my sisters came by occasionally to visit Mother. I had expected some regular assistance with Mother's care, but that was not to be. They had varying degrees of personal problems and other commitments, and that just was as it was. I'll speak more on siblings in the chapter on families.

Driving

When I arrived in Indy, Mother was driving fine, per normal, and without any sign of a problem. She was a calm and careful driver to begin with, and that had not changed.

For a number of years before his death, Dad had deferred the driving to Mother. First of all, he was too easily distracted, and it was common for him to turn around and talk to us in the back seat while he was driving. Of course, we were pretty quick to say, "Dad, watch the road!" And he would reply, "I am. I am," as though he had it all under control. He was also more nervous when he got excited. Other times, he could be having a conversation with himself or someone else, present or not; we could tell this not just by his speaking out loud but also he acted out all the facial expressions as well. He didn't answer himself in those self-conversations, so we probably thought it was harmless, except when he was driving.

I don't remember his putting up any struggle about giving up the wheel. I wasn't living in town at the time, so I don't know the particulars. Some of my sisters said they wouldn't ride in a car with him driving. That was understandable. Anyway, Mother took the wheel, and not just for the town and local trip driving.

Mother and Dad "trailered" for a dozen years after he retired in the early 1970s. She did most of their driving when they took many trailer trips. Driving a station wagon from the 1970s that was a boat in itself, they also had a substantial trailer attached. They sent me a photo of the whole rig when they were at some stop in the Arizona desert, and the car/trailer combo looked like a train about a half block long.

On one cross-country excursion, they drove to Pasadena for the Rose Bowl and also stayed up all night the previous night to get good seats for the Rose parade. They also joined a trailer caravan that went deep into Mexico for a few weeks. They did like adventure.

Mother and Dad flew to Mexico for a couple of winters instead of making the standard trek to Florida. I had recommended a few locations to them. Merida and the Yucatan Peninsula were one area; Mazatlan was another. They especially enjoyed Merida.

They were also involved in Elderhostel. That was a new option whereby retirees went to various universities, and attended a mini-university session while visiting local spots of historic and natural beauty. One of the Elderhostel sessions was in Montreal; another was in South Carolina; and an extended session was in England and Ireland.

The hardest and most dangerous of the driving conditions they were in was the trip up Pike's Peak in Colorado. Mother told me she would never, ever, ever drive that again. I believe it was a two-lane road then, and they were inches from a very steep drop off the mountain road. At one point they had to back up to let another car come down, and that was pretty scary as well. Dad probably had cigarettes in both hands and was yelling, "Look out! Look out!" As I said before, two wars, especially Korea, and a plethora of other stressors had taken a toll on his nervous system. Of course many people are that nervous without even having gone to war.

So, Mother's driving had been proven by many years, many kids in the car, and the challenge of the road up Pike's Peak. She still stayed calm and drove.

Bernice's problems with driving after her AD diagnosis began with directions or route to take. She knew the locations. She knew where she wanted to go, and she drove very well. However, she began to forget how to get where she wanted to go. She had probably kept this problem from me for a while by eventually finding where she wanted or needed to drive. At this stage, she only drove to half a dozen locations, and never had a problem I knew of. She'd been to those places so often that she could go on auto pilot. I rode with her at least weekly in order to see that she was driving okay. I didn't want to rush in and take the keys from her; enough was being taken from her already. Nor did I say I was testing her; I just casually asked if she would mind driving when we were going somewhere.

Then came the day when she had to tell me about a driving problem, and I was so proud of her when she did. She asked, "Heydon, would you please drive me to the hairdresser?"

"Sure," I replied, without asking the reason.

After a moment she added, "I just don't remember how to get there." It was a few miles away through some twists and turns and off the main street. She probably would have kept that new memory loss secret, but she had a scheduled appointment so she couldn't gamble on finding the place eventually; and, after all, the hairdresser is something she wouldn't want to miss!

"I'll be happy to take you anywhere you want to go," I added. So, we handled that stage, and it made me feel good that we could talk about it.

On our trips to the hairdresser—a lady who had her shop attached to her house—I would go in and find out when Mother would be finished. The hairdresser was someone Mother had gone to for years and knew of Mother's memory problem. She also knew that I was looking after Bernice. The hairdresser and the customers in various stages of perms or dryers would look at me with some admiration, and that would bolster my self-image for the day.

Mother still drove well. Then one afternoon she drove to see my sister a few miles away. She stayed longer than planned, and dusk was turning to darkness. I called and said that I would drive up, and she could follow me home. I felt that night driving might be unsafe for her now. We started home, and soon I turned left onto a four-lane divided highway. She was behind me, driving fine, had her turn signal on, but she turned too soon and into the two lanes of oncoming traffic. Those lanes were stopped since their light was red. She quickly saw what she'd done, backed up and then followed me the rest of the way home.

When we arrived home, I said, "I think it's better if you don't do any more night driving. It can be pretty confusing out there." She agreed, and that was that.

A few months later, she drove to a medical appointment at her doctor's office. When she'd been gone an hour and a half, I received a call from a fellow at a service station near the doctor's office. He asked me if Bernice Buchanan was my mother. I replied that she was, and then he said she was standing there with him and was having trouble finding her car in the parking lot.

I spoke with Mother, told her to wait exactly where she was, and then told the station attendant that I would be up there right away to get her. I picked her up, drove across the street to the parking lot, found the car and then had her follow me home.

She was laughing about the incident, seeing it as a simple bit of confusion. I was very concerned because when I learned that she was at the service station, I knew that she had had to walk across a very busy, dangerous intersection. At that point, I gently said, "I'll drive you to the doctor's office from now on." She agreed, though she said it wasn't necessary.

That left only one location she was driving to—church. She might be able to cut back on her volunteer work there during the week, but she still had to go to service on Sundays. I drove down with her to see how she handled it, and she was okay. So, I said all right. Part of this was because I knew she wouldn't give up attending church, and I wasn't a regular church attendee.

A few weeks later she was telling me about church when she returned home one Sunday. She casually mentioned taking a wrong turn on the way to church and had gone an alternate route. Somehow I knew right then that the safest thing would be for her to stop driving altogether at that point.

Starting the following Sunday, I went to church with her on a regular basis. I still let her drive once more just to gauge her awareness and reflexes; I wondered how she would do in an emergency situation. However, from then on I drove her everywhere, and she didn't complain.

In April 1994, we were driving along one day, and Mother brought up the subject of renewing her driver's license. I thought she had forgotten about that. So I said, "You really don't need to. I can take you anywhere you want to go." She quickly deferred to my judgment and said, "Okay." So that was probably her last thought—and certainly our last conversation—about driving. I believe we transitioned through giving up the wheel far easier and safer than so many other cases I've heard of. We did it bit by bit, and she was able to keep her dignity without a radical command that she couldn't drive any more. Admittedly, giving up the wheel is easier for someone if they know that they always have a ready driver.

Health Care Representative (HCR)

After I began driving Mother to the doctor, I would stay in the waiting room while she had her appointment. She started having trouble remembering what the doctor had said, so she asked me to come into the consultation with her. I developed a working relationship with her doctor and nurse. I became her unofficial advocate and never thought to formalize it with official designation.

In mid-1994, Mother and I were watching a show on PBS which had a brief reference to respirators and life support. When she saw a patient in bed hooked up with tubes and machines, she suddenly spoke up and said, "I wouldn't want that."

At that point I said, "Then we better speak with your doctor and find out what choices you have." I didn't try to talk her out of respirators and such because I felt the same way about it for myself.

Her doctor spoke to her privately to determine her understanding of life support but more importantly to determine if she was able to make that decision on her own. Even then, he assessed her competence since it is a serious decision. Then he learned from her that she wanted me to make her health care decisions whenever the need arose.

I was called into the examining room, and the doctor explained what was happening. He interviewed and evaluated me. Then, I agreed to be her Health Care Representative (HCR), and we completed the paperwork.

Like many people, I assumed that the patient's doctor would automatically respect the family's choice in the patient's medical treatment when the patient was judged incompetent and had not made out an Advance Directive. I thought this would be especially true in the matter of resuscitation and artificial life support. However, there can be a lot of gray area here. The first questions might be "What does 'family's choice' signify? Would that be a majority or plurality vote or…?" I can understand the quandary of a physician in dealing with this.

The best way to avoid being placed on machinery and mechanisms for artificially extending your life is to create a Living Will while you are still competent; appoint someone you trust as your HCR; complete the necessary paperwork for Living Will and HCR; and discuss your wishes with your family, HCR, and physician. You should be able to obtain the appropriate forms in your doctor's office. That's where my wife and I completed our individual forms.

If a patient has an HCR or guardian, that person can make medical decisions for the patient when the patient is unable to do so directly. However, guardianship is a legal process that must be delegated by a judge. Actually, the choices for life extension can be far more complicated than simply choosing life support or not. There are the additional choices of food, hydration, machinery, resuscitation and others. I'll cover that in more detail in chapter nine.

There are two final notes on this matter. Once you have completed the paperwork for your Living Will and HCR, make sure that your doctor's office has placed their copies in your medical record and reassess the situation annually. I filled out my forms five years ago, and the doctor's office—a busy HMO—made a copy to put in my records there. When I spoke with my doctor's nurse last month about the protocol for Living Wills and HCRs, she added that there was no copy of a Living Will or HCR designation in my medical records. That's scary. I filled out my forms in that office; they notarized the forms; and they made a copy to place in my records five years ago. Although I have the original copies in a secure place and my wife knew of their existence, she may not have found them during a most stressful life-and-death period. What if something had happened to my wife in the meantime? My fate would be left to the state law applying to someone without record of medical Advance Directive, and that is something I would never wish to have; that could mean long-term existence on a respirator and a feeding tube surgically implanted into my body.

Last month, soon after finding that the Living Will and HCR forms were missing from my medical records, there was also a national reminder of the importance of these medical designations. A family in Florida was in an emotionally wrenching battle about the future of Mrs. Schiavo—a young lady who had been on a respirator for many years and had tube feeding as well. She had never completed a Living Will or HCR designation form. There were polarizing attitudes in the country about what should or should not have been done in her treatment. The U.S. President and Congress were intervening inappropriately, and it was a horrible mess. The majority of U.S. citizens did agree that government should not get involved in what was a family matter. However, on the family level, there was still serious and unresolved disagreement.

I can't stress enough how important it is to complete your Advance Directive. Further, find a dependable HCR—someone you trust to make the most important medical decisions about your life when you are incapable of making them yourself. Be sure to speak with your family, HCR, and doctor about this. Then, make sure a copy of each form is in your medical records. If you doubt the seriousness of the matter or think you're too young for this to apply, research the Schiavo family case online or at your library.

Townhouse Office

One day I went into the administration office of the complex to report a problem with the dishwasher. I had been in a couple of other times to report other maintenance problems—things that Mother may not notice, or that she might have trouble explaining to the office, or that she might not even bother to have corrected. This time the manager said, "If you're going to be living there and reporting any maintenance needs, your name should be on the lease as well." She was telling me indirectly that they really didn't have to listen to me as an outsider. So, Mother thought that adding me to the lease was a good idea, and it was done. It satisfied the office so that I could speak officially for the unit, and the manager also had a second person on the lease as being responsible for the rent being paid.

Church

Going to church on Sunday morning was an unspoken commandment for my parents. After Dad's death, it continued so for Bernice. However, it was a commandment that she put upon herself, and she did it with great love. The church, with its sanctuary, choir, friends and familial embrace, provided her with much joy. By her actions and attitude she had fully incorporated the Christian mantra, "Whenever two or more are gathered in my name, there is love."

Church was her fountain of refreshment, her point of reference, and her personal reserve to help face the tough trials that life had to offer. More importantly, she lived her beliefs day in and day out—the schedule of 24/7 as is so often used in today's parlance. The institution was a chance to recharge her batteries with other people in a sacred yet joyful atmosphere. I say recharge because the direction, purpose, and basic strength were already in her essential nature.

We children were required to attend Sunday school. That was a commandment. Then, we often went to church as well. As children, we were not as excited about these mandatory Sunday church activities as our parents were.

Speaking of church, I'm reminded of our having had a blessing before every meal at home. That was never forgotten. We would always have our daily supper at 6 PM. And, as one of my sisters said at the memorial, Mother would always have a warm, nutritious meal ready for all of us.

The first church I remember attending was the First Baptist Church of Tampa. I was five when we started there. For the most part, we just attended Sunday school. Occasionally, the Sunday school class made an excursion away from the church. Once we visited a Catholic church. Another time we visited a Jewish Temple. We were always welcomed, and had a nice experience in seeing the environments where other people worshipped.

On another occasion, the Sunday school class had a field trip to the park across the street from the church—Plant Park, I believe—and bought peanuts to feed the pigeons. That park borders the Hillsborough River and is across the river from downtown Tampa. Being outdoors was the best of Sunday schools—seeing the natural work of God.

Our next-door neighbors—an elderly couple—attended First Baptist and gave us a ride. Mother went with us and attended early church while we were in Sunday school.

Dad attended a Methodist church where he taught Sunday school and also sang in the choir. After our Sunday school, we would go to pick him up and then sometimes go to that church for their service. I'm not sure why we were at different churches except that Dad really enjoyed and related to the minister at Palma Ceil Methodist. It was a smaller church and exceptionally friendly.

When we moved to Lakeland, we joined another Methodist church. Six years later, when we moved back to Indiana, we again joined a Methodist church. After being in Indiana for six years, my parents joined a neighborhood Presbyterian congregation. It proved to be a comfortable "church home" for them—congregation and minister seemed inspired and inspiring. As usual, my parents contributed a lot of themselves to the church of which we were members.

Dad felt the same as Mother in terms of the Sunday church ritual. His was not a serene approach to life as Mother's was, since he was a very exuberant and extroverted person. He loved to sing and did so in the choir of every church we belonged to. Also, he would start singing spontaneously as we walked down the street, and I don't just mean humming a favorite hymn. He would bellow out, "He leadeth me, He leadeth me...!" or one of another twenty or so of his favorites.

Part of my father's joy in that free expression was probably related to his recent arrival back from the war in Korea. He had survived.

Now the war and killing cold were far away, and he was safe at home with his family, and in the warm, semi-tropical climate of central Florida. It was 1953, and Tampa was still a casual little city with a relatively small population and plenty of space to roam. He had just turned forty years old, and the world seemed wonderful. Frankly, he had a lot to sing about.

*****

Bernice Buchanan was a Christian in my eyes, and the truest example I've known. She incorporated the principles of Christ into her life, and she taught them to her children. "Do unto others as you would have others do unto you." "Love one another, as I have loved you." "Whatever you do to the least of these, you do to me." And there were many more.

Mother lived her religion but never spoke about it. She didn't define herself with regard to religion or denomination or individual church. Through a lifetime of practice, Bernice had found and lived by what worked for her. She was always in touch with a "Higher Power." She didn't care what anyone else's religion was. We were not raised with any prejudice toward other people's religion or color or nationality or whatever. The only exception to that which comes to mind was a prejudice against mean or obnoxious people. Even then, she didn't vocally say anything about mean people; however, when an example was in immediate view, she would ever so slightly shake her head to illustrate that this was not acceptable behavior.

Mother taught us the lessons, but that is not to say we absorbed all of them or demonstrated all of them when we were out of her presence. However, for the most part, I believe they stuck pretty well. I have watched my siblings in action with all different manner of human beings over the years and have never witnessed any prejudice by them toward others, or any dishonesty.

I never heard Bernice say a bad word about another human being. I never heard her yell. I never heard her use one word of profanity. And those qualities are just the start really. I did hear her say "Darn" a few times. Even then, the word was directed toward something she had done herself, unhappy with a sewing seam or perhaps she overcooked a vegetable.

A few years ago, I was visiting childhood friends in Tampa. At the home of one, his mother, a true Southern lady, gave me a hug and said in her very melodious accent, "Heydie Bu, how are you doing?"

"Fine, Mrs. Miller," I replied.

"And how is your mutha?"

"Good. Her short-term memory is going away, but her smile and loving nature are still there," I answered.

Then Mrs. Miller turned to her visiting neighbor and said, "Heydon grew up down the street from us. He and Bobby have been friends since they were six. His mutha, Bernice Buchanan, is such a gentle lady. I saw her raise five children and didn't raise her voice one time. I never saw anything like it. It was amazing."

So, that's the way Mother was, and the impression really stuck with people.

Volunteer Service

As an extension of her religion, Mother was selfless. Not only did she provide endlessly for her husband and five children, she also gave a great deal to her church and the community. She helped in whatever the church needed, from the sewing circle to the soup kitchen. In the community, she helped at least weekly at the Red Cross by teaching blind ladies how to sew and do macramé. One of my prized possessions is the ten-year service pin from the Red Cross in recognition of her volunteer work. The pin is of no value financially, but it signifies one example of her selfless service.

Wherever she went, this gentle soul was loved. One of the blind ladies, also named Bernice, would call Mother for advice on this or that. Once it was to tell Mother about a new fellow she was dating; he was blind also. I could tell the two Bernice's were of similar natures because of the way Mother would laugh and giggle with her on the phone. They were like two schoolgirls sharing simple joys. Whenever I picked up the phone first, the blind Bernice would tell me how much Mother meant to her, how much she loved her.

*****

The founder of Mother's religion said, "If you would enter the kingdom of Heaven, you must be like little children." And that was one of her traits—she carried the wide-eyed wonder and innocence of a child, a being with neither guile nor malice toward any other person.

*****

After finishing high school, I didn't share much of my parents' church experience. College, the army, travels, and living in New York and Los Angeles distanced me physically for the next twenty-five years of my life. While home on leave or vacation, I would go to a church service with my folks, but that was the extent of our shared church experience at that point.

When Dad passed away, and I returned home, I began to go sporadically to Sunday church service with Mother. When she could no longer drive, we went together every Sunday since I was her driver. It was pleasant, and we always sat in the same pew and most often the same seats. All of the regular people seemed to sit in their same seats. It was part of the natural order of things.

Then Mother lost track of what day it was. She became worried that she would miss church. Many weekday mornings I would see her laying out her favorite dress. When I asked why she had it on the bed, she said that she was getting ready for church. Other times, she would ask me in the morning, "Heydon, what day is it?" Or, "Is today Sunday?" She was at the point where calendars with written appointments and family birthdays served no purpose because she had no point of reference. She didn't know one day from the next. Everything was running together.

With a certain amount of guilt, I should admit something here. One Sunday morning I was feeling very tired and didn't feel like going to church or anywhere. Per usual, Mother asked me what day it was. "Saturday," I said. "Tomorrow is church day." It pacified her, especially feeling that she hadn't missed it. By later in the day, she would forget it altogether. I don't lie and especially didn't want to do that to Mother, but I just didn't feel good that day; and I couldn't tell her no without truly disappointing her. That only happened once.

Another worry would suddenly pop up when Bernice thought she didn't have anything to wear to church. This was not the concern of a shallow person who wished for a more stylish dress. This was the frustration of a gracious lady who couldn't find her dress, who couldn't differentiate one dress from another as the dresses hung next to each other in her closet. This was part of her neurological disintegration. A similar frustration—and one that is shared by many AD patients—was when she would say, "I don't have any money." It's not that she would say that after checking her wallet or purse; often, the phrase just popped out. I tried to reassure her that she did have money, but the level of emotional discomfort that brought up the money fear would also not allow any of my reassurance to get through to comfort her. Eventually, I asked the POA to make a list of Mother's assets so I could show Mother that she did have money. Still, that was only a temporary pacifier.

Sometimes Nancy and Pat would go to church with us. We were a happy foursome. Nancy, Pat, and I would often spark off of Mother's joy. We continued going to church after I had taken Bernice to a facility. I would ask the nursing home aides to have her ready at a certain time, then pick her up and go. When her infirmity increased, it was very slow walking from the parking lot to the church. Then, it became even more complicated with the wheelchair—picking her up at the nursing home and storing the wheelchair in the back of my truck. Then, incontinence set in, and that was another complication.

A couple members of the church used to visit her monthly in the nursing home. They would visit various people at home or in nursing facilities. I always appreciated that a great deal. These two ladies knew how special Mother's character was, and didn't mind that Bernice couldn't recognize them. They always saw her smiling heart, and the way she greeted them with love. At Easter, the church would send Mother a blooming lily also.

I made it a point to take some fresh produce from the garden to those two ladies as a little thank you for their visits to see Mother. Beyond that, I took boxes of fresh tomatoes for the soup kitchen's use at that church. When some church members started their own gardens on the land next to the church, I tilled some plots to help get them started. These little deeds were all done in appreciation for the two ladies who visited Bernice.

*****

By a twist of fate, I was temporarily working at Mother's church four years after she entered the nursing home. I worked on a medical research project which used her church as one of their study sites. This was a very innovative project attempting to train the elderly in memory techniques in order to help them stay independent as long as possible. As a memory trainer, I taught a five-week class in these techniques. I loved it, and the students had a great time, too. The participants had to be over sixty-five, and free of dementia when they entered the program.

One day after class I was walking to my truck when a few of Mother's church friends noticed me in the parking lot. We said hellos, and they asked how Mother was doing.

"We sure miss seeing you and your mother in church. Every Sunday you were there in your regular spots, as were we," said one of the ladies. It's interesting how people gravitate toward a regular seat at church.

"Your parents made such a fine couple," said the other lady. "And your father had such presence."

"Yes," I said, "he was one-of-a-kind."

"Yes," she quickly replied, "the special kind."

I couldn't help but wonder if that was an old crush she had on Dad. However, one thing was certain—each of my parents had presence in their own very different styles. Also, they were a notable couple in looks, character and achievement.

Helping Care Recipient with Personal Hygiene

During the descent of Alzheimer's disease (AD), patients eventually reach the point at which they can no longer take care of their personal hygiene or dress themselves. Those conditions will produce an extra challenge for the caregiver—additional stressors that the caregiver may not be prepared for. Since it can be difficult to stay on top of the care recipient's current needs, anticipating additional patient decline is not generally a priority. Pondering the new duties of handling incontinence, bathing, and dressing may be overwhelming.

Some physical, psychological, and emotional strain may well be faced by caregiver and care recipient when the intimate ADLs (Activities of Daily Living) begin. Yet more stressors will be added when the caregiver and care recipient are of different sexes. There is the social taboo of adult children and parents of different genders seeing one another without clothes. In AD caregiving, it means the adult child seeing the parent without clothes.

The matter of cleaning up the care recipient—regardless of the patient's gender—involves another intimacy frowned on by society. I don't remember anticipating these tasks in advance. As I wrote earlier, the demands of daily caregiving don't allow much time for such contemplation of the future. Of course, there are matters that I probably just couldn't—or didn't want to—think about. Handling personal hygiene and dressing would be two of those areas. Taking Mother to a nursing home would be another.

While recently reviewing my journal from the caregiving years, I found one note on this subject which read "Call Central Indiana Council on Aging for assistance in bathing Mother."

*****

Concerning the adult child-parent/different gender matter, the common caregiving scenario is a daughter taking care of her father. This arrangement is less noticed by society for at least a couple of reasons. Historically, women have done the bulk of nursing and emotional nurturing, so that vision has been placed in our heads. Second, the majority of caregivers now are women, so statistics alone give some psychological acceptance of daughter-Father caregiving.

The adult son-Mother caregiving situation is fairly new and uncommon. At least initially, it could be very stressful for both caregiver and care recipient. Since there is no measurable correlation between the level of dementia and incontinence, the care recipient could be very aware when the situation calls for the required intimacy.

My mother and I had not discussed this matter as the dementia increased. Bernice was very private and modest, and probably would have been quite disturbed for me to see her without clothes; however, she would have been more disturbed—not to mention brokenhearted—if I had sentenced her to a nursing home because I didn't want to handle the hygiene task. It was bound to be stressful either way, and for a while I felt like a pioneer in uncharted lands.

Part of the quandary was handled for us. Please bear with me as I wind through this. Mother had a Transient Ischemic Attack (TIA), spent three days in the hospital, and then her doctor ordered her to a convalescent center with orders for 24-hour care. During my daily visits, she would constantly ask for me to take her home. I would reply that we had to wait for the doctor's okay. After a few minutes, she would again ask me to take her home. She only needed unskilled, 24-hour care at that point, so I formulated a plan. I brought the physical and occupational therapists home to evaluate exactly what Bernice's needs were in the home environment. Once I had their report, I rearranged furniture and made necessary alterations to make Mother's living environment as comfortable and functional as possible.

I contacted a homecare agency that had been recommended and worked with the agency owner in making a homecare plan. As a result, I hired home health aides (HHA) for twelve hours a day; and I covered the other twelve hours of the day. All of those aides were female since it was most important at that point. The cost for HHAs was totally out of pocket as neither Medicare nor Bernice's private health insurance would cover any costs for "unskilled" needs.

With everything in place, I went to Bernice's physician and explained the plan and all preparations made. He agreed to allow Mother to come home. She was happy as could be. With the HHAs covering twelve hours each day, I was able to avoid the hygiene and dressing issues for a little while. They would dress her for bed before they left each night and also take her to the bathroom. Bernice was cautious about taking liquids at night, so she wouldn't have to get up for the bathroom. Also, they bathed her during the day.

One evening, near midnight, I woke to rustling noises coming from her bedroom. I thought she was tossing and turning, and I waited for her to go back to sleep. The tossing continued. I got up and went into her room.

"Are you having trouble sleeping?" I asked.

"Yes," she replied.

I noticed she kept pulling at the plastic cover over her brief. She knew where her discomfort was, but she didn't know what it was or how to fix it. I then checked the brief and found it was wet.

"Oh, no," I thought. The dreaded moment had arrived. There was no way around it. Nor was there any time to dwell on it.

"Okay," I said, "we need to change that brief, and then you'll be fine."

"Okay," she answered.

There was low light in the room with only a plug-in night light and some indirect light from the hall. She hadn't really acknowledged who I was, and may have thought she was dreaming.

I changed her as the aides had instructed me and could tell she was already more comfortable without that wet agitation. Then I stood up, tucked her covers up to her neck, gave her a kiss on the forehead, and said, "Sleep tight, and don't let the bedbugs bite." That was something she used to say to us as kids. Now she smiled, and I turned to go back to my room. I was still a little unsettled about what had just happened. As I reached the door, I heard her voice from behind.

"Thank you. Thank you," she said in a low, sincere tone.

"You're very welcome," I answered.

That was my first episode of cleaning and changing. Her note of thanks, and the tone that carried so much gratitude, helped me get over the uncommon experience. Changing and cleaning became easier with each episode.

Over time, my view on the cleaning and changing process evolved to different perspectives. Initially, I had recognized the patient as my mother, and someone who had done a lot for me. Later, I saw her as a great person who had done a lot to make a better world. Finally, while handling the cleaning and changing, I simply saw her as a human being in need of assistance.

Several years after completing my home caregiving, I read an account of Mother Teresa and her role in helping people. More importantly, I read of her perception in doing hands-on care; that is, she recognized Christ in every person she helped. I could understand that view through the changing perceptions I experienced in helping my mother. In this process, my task was much easier because Bernice was already the closest figure to Christ that I had ever known or known of.

In the end, I decided that the matter of helping a loved one with their personal hygiene needs was reduced to two simple components—action and attitude. The action is cleaning and changing a patient. The attitude is hopefully one of love. Also, I realized that pondering the earlier-mentioned psychological and emotional difficulties would have been pointless. Once a caregiver is fully committed to a loved one, all other issues (i.e., modesty, taboos, etc.) become meaningless. If you love that person—that soul—you do what needs to be done to keep them healthy, clean, and comfortable—period.

Consider the role Mothers have served throughout history in keeping us clean. Further, when I think of the family caregivers who have handled all the needs—especially personal hygiene—of severely disabled children all of their lives, I am in awe of them. Mine was a very small part in the scale of things but enough to appreciate those people who have sacrificed their whole lives to it, and enough to understand the well of love a caregiver can also tap in to.

Mother had probably changed a million diapers for me, so it was no big deal if I had to change some for her. We simply have to do what's necessary and overcome the taboos that society throws our way. I was able to bypass the full-bathing and dressing issues. The outside aides could do that during their shift. I was thankful for that.

If I reach an old age where a diaper is necessary, I do have a different wish. As I've told friends lightheartedly since the caregiving experience, "I don't mind if I have to wear a diaper or brief some day. After all, how much difference is there between a diaper and an Indian dhoti? I just hope to be able to change the garment myself."

Gardening—Food, Flowers, and Therapy

Gardens were the last thing on my mind when I made the decision to move back to Indiana. Everything was too serious at that point. However, gardening turned out to be a great activity that Mother and I could share as her mind slipped away. Further, it turned out to be a priceless therapeutic tool for me during my caregiving years.

It was the beginning of spring, 1992. Selma came by our home to visit one day and said, "Bernice, my church is renting garden plots again this year. Why don't you and Heydon take one?"

Mother started, "Well..." and looked to me for an answer. I said, "Yes." I was full of enthusiasm but lacking in experience. Growing some basil in pots was about the depth of my gardening knowledge.

We had a 20'x40' garden, and the rent was $20 for the season. I did the tilling and other heavy preparation. Then Mother joined for the planting. It was wonderful to watch this gentle old woman put the seedlings in their new home and pat the earth around them, as though she were tucking in a child for the night. She even hummed, and I could have

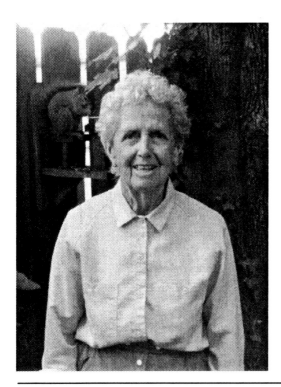

Spring, 1991
Mother enjoyed
the back patio
and the wildlife.
Our guest squirrel
is having lunch
behind her.

Circa 1991
Another baby
looks to Bernice
for comfort.

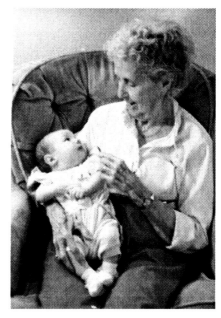

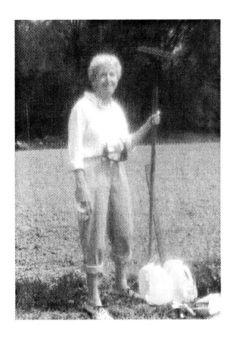

Spring, 1992
Bernice is anxious to
begin planting in the
freshly-tilled garden.

This photo was out of
focus, but I include it
to show her zeal for
the garden and work.

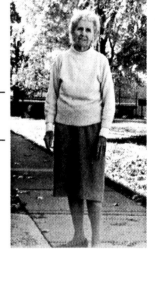

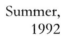

Summer,
1992

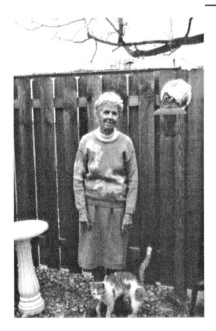

Fall, 1992
Neighbor came
to visit, or at
least be
scratched.

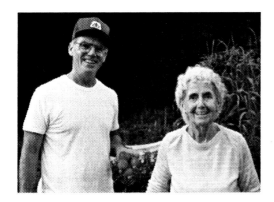
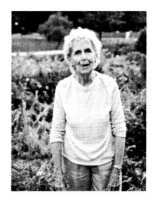

1993 summer garden finds us once again growing healthy
food, talking about family history, and having fun.

Fall, 1993
Nancy and
Bernice are
wearing their
new pepper
necklaces—the
latest fashion
by Heydon—
and holding
bowls of
flowers.
We all got a
kick out of it!

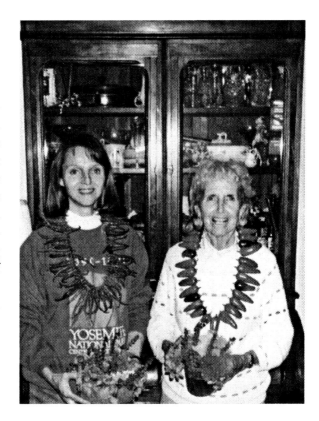

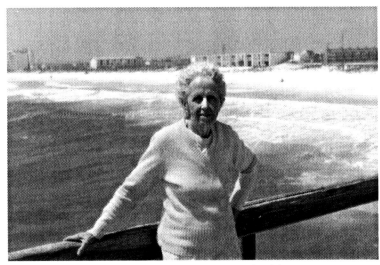

April, 1994, Gulf Coast, Florida
The day before our return to Indiana—the drive which
included the sudden and horrendous "Catastrophic Effect"
as described in chapter seven. It was Alzheimer's disease
at its absolutely most terrifying.

Summer, 1995
Our last garden
together, and the
Mammoth Russian
sunflowers share it
with us.
Note the cinch
belt on Bernice's
waist. We used it
for support to
keep her from fal-
ling at that point.

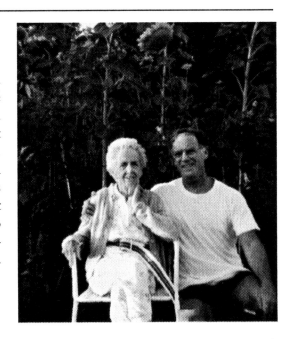

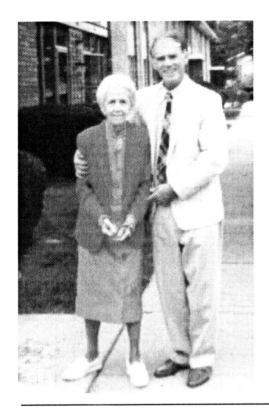

Summer, 1995
Sunday Church Day.
Mother found
remarkable comfort
in worship shared
with others.
Though always
cheerful, Sunday
church service was
the most joyful time
of her week.

Fall, 1995
Another church day.
During her last six
months at home,
Alzheimer's was
showing more of
the physical
deterioration.

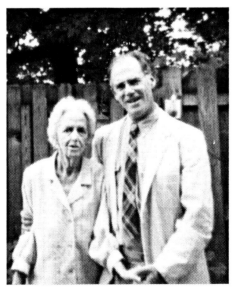

sworn it was a lullaby. After she bedded the plants, I would christen them with a little water from Walden Pond, a souvenir from my visit to Henry Thoreau's happy abode.

After a while she said, "Grandma Pet would sure have loved this garden. She really enjoyed working outdoors. Heydon, I wish you could have met her. She was so much fun." Sometimes I thought Grandma Pet influenced my mother more than her own parents had. Special treatment is not uncommon from a grandparent, especially for a solitary granddaughter, not to mention that Pet's only child had been a son. As we worked day after day, Mother told me more about her family—grandparents, parents, and siblings.

As we worked in the garden, I reflected on the nearby garden plot my parents had rented a few years back. I could still look over and see my father working in the garden. Working intensely in the hot sun, he talked to himself a lot, often in animated terms, oblivious to anyone around him. At that particular moment he happened to be revisiting World War II. He spoke to the tall corn stalks, as though they were junior officers standing at ease in the light wind.

"I told General Clark [Mark Clark] that was the wrong move!" The stalks of corn were lined up in formation and were obediently quiet as my father continued with a shrug of his shoulders, "But what can you do. He was the Commanding General." Dad had been on the tactical advisory staff of General Mark Clark as the allied forces crossed Sicily and then up the mainland of Italy during the Italian campaign of World War II.

One day I brought a young lady to the garden to help us. She was my girlfriend, later my fiancée, now my wife. Nancy and Mother enjoyed each other from the start. Toward the end of the season, as the mid-September sun began to soften, I made big necklaces for each of them out of various red chili peppers and garlands of fresh flowers for their hair. I anointed them as "Queen Mother" and "Princess-in-Waiting." What a picture they made! When they smiled for the camera, I could feel the spirit of Grandma Pet running through us and binding us all together in the merriment.

We had other visitors in the garden that summer—friends and family members who came to look and chat. This was our outdoor classroom—an open forum that also produced healthy food and beautiful flowers—for us, and the other people with whom we shared them.

*****

One of my sisters came by one day when I was at the garden alone. She looked at the garden, smiled, and said, "Isn't God wonderful?"

"Yes," I happily agreed, "we make a good team."

"What do you mean?" she asked suspiciously.

"Well," I replied, "we do our part. He does His part. And we end up with this." I pointed to the healthy and fruitful plants.

"No, Heydon," she answered with some acidity, "God did it ALL!"

ALL? I thought to myself, "That's interesting. That means Mother and I have wasted a lot of time and some money by buying seeds, germinating them at home to get an early start on the season, transplanting them to this garden, watering them regularly, feeding them, and weeding them. And she's saying we didn't have to do any of that to get this wonderful garden." I was going to mention this to my sister, but I decided to try another approach to get through to her.

"If God did it all," I started, "then I guess He loves us twice as much as He loves the gardener in the plot next to us."

"What do you mean?" she asked testily.

"Well, we have the same type and number of plants as our neighbor. However, we have twice as many tomatoes as he does."

She couldn't think to reply and just said, "Oh, forget it!" Uh-oh, I could see trouble brewing. This attitude was the second incident to remind me of her lingering issues. I was becoming the target for some-one's unhappiness. I mention this occurrence because it was a preview of the sibling conflict soon to come in the matter of parental caregiving. I began to believe that she really wasn't well. However, I brushed off the incident as though it were nothing. I wouldn't let anything interfere with the joy that Mother and I shared in nurturing that garden.

*****

After that garden, Mother and I had two more years of gardens together. The disability and confusion of dementia began to take its toll. Even as her strength began to wane, Mother wanted to help. When planting became too hard for her, she would switch to pulling out little weeds that grew around the seedlings. Toward the end, when we went to the garden, I would carry a comfortable chair for her to sit in the shade of a nearby oak while I gardened on.

Finally, she could only sit in the car, as we drove to the garden so she could see the progress. I watched her as she watched the garden. I had learned so much from her in terms of style—working with love and nurturing the plants like beloved children who depend on you to help with so many of their needs—feeding them, protecting them from harm, and simply conveying the true feelings of care and concern. Mother looked at the plants, then turned to me with a smile, and said, "Looks pretty good." That was our last garden together.

After closing the apartment, I moved to my new home. There was some open land in the back, and I plowed a new garden which I've worked every year since. It's a quiet spot surrounded by tall, swaying trees; and I've always felt that Mother is there as well, guiding me to make the right moves. At times, I also have the sense that Grandma Pet is with us, too.

On Bernice's second Mother's Day at the nursing home, I told her about the year's new plants—potatoes, sweet peas, various types of tomatoes, Brussels sprouts, corn, zucchini, basil, and many flowers. She listened, nodded and smiled. Finally, I left and then felt melancholy— a sadness that she couldn't be out there again with me on that warm spring afternoon.

I pulled into my parking spot at the back of the house and climbed out of the truck. A movement registered at the side of my eye. I looked out at the fence supports for the sweet peas. About six feet from me a baby grackle sat on the fence pole, wobbling back and forth. I thought, "Funny, that bird's not afraid of me. It's not flying away." The baby bird stared at me curiously. Then the mother flew up and sat next to it. She stared at me briefly, but she wasn't curious. Through some signal, she conveyed the need to take off, and the baby was off again for an unstable, ten-foot flight. I watched for a while, as the Mother prodded and taught the little bird what to do from runway to runway.

At that point I realized the unity of it all. I felt in step with that prehistoric and perpetual life process–a parent guiding the offspring. Mother had shared her knowledge with me—knowledge of the garden, family and life; now this mama grackle guided her chick in new skills.

There was nothing to be sad about. We learn. We work. We teach. We love. We move on. Mother's spirit has stayed with me in the garden, especially her smile and laughter. Good things never die.

*****

From what I've read and experienced, many AD patients keep their memory problem secret as long as possible. Why? Probably due to a fear that they'll be put away in "the poor house" (the older generation's term) or nursing home. This could be coupled with the fear that no one loves them enough to take care of them at home, or that their loved ones have other priorities and won't care for them. Or, it could just be an overwhelming sense of vulnerability and despair to feel your mind beginning to disintegrate.

In Mother's case, I found various writings around the townhouse that showed parts of her process of mental loss. Previously, she had an evenly-round, flowing script with perfect spelling. Now, there were the examples of handwriting with the etched, angled letters of stop-start handwriting; then a scrap paper with "Margy or Margie" written in that uncertain mode as though writing both names might help her to remember which one is right; then a note to her brother and sister-in-law that grew increasingly scribbled as she got to the end. She finished that note but had set it aside and forgot to mail it. It read, "Dear Bernard & Evelyn, All is well here. Heydon takes care of most everything around, so I take it easy. The girls come and go. Hope all is well with you all. Have a Merry Christmas. Write sometime. Love, Bernice." (end of note) That was written in December 1993. It was painful for me to see those handwriting attempts because I could feel some of the anxiety she was going through. Her logic was still intact, but her dexterity was slipping away. The neurological disability was growing from memory loss to diminished physical skills. This must have been frightening for Mother and even worse for Alzheimer's patients who lived alone.

CHAPTER 5

FAMILIES AT THE CROSSROADS

All happy families are alike; every unhappy family is
unhappy in its own way.
    —Leo Tolstoy, *Anna Karenina*

To put the family in order, we must first cultivate our
personal life; we must first set our hearts right.
    —Confucius

In matters of conscience, the law of majority has no place.
    —Gandhi

One loyal friend is better than ten thousand family
members.
    —Unknown

FAMILY HEALTH, STRENGTH, AND SOLIDARITY CAN FACE NO
greater challenge than the issue of caregiving for a beloved, widowed parent with terminal dementia. In this case, I refer to adult children helping their mother through her burden of Alzheimer's disease. When the time comes to face this most serious of issues, a person may well discover that the traditional concept of family is truly an illusion.

*****

This chapter is divided into several portions. The first is a discussion of family itself; then the issue of family caregivers; then the matter of solitary caregivers; and, finally, the process of choosing or avoiding parental caregiving. For those readers who would prefer to skip the discussion of family dynamics in caregiving, you can move on to chapter six.

What is a Family?

I bring up this question and subsequent discussion based on an experience I had early in my caregiving years. One of my sisters said to me privately, "Heydon, I don't want to shock you, but I believe that you and I are the only ones willing to work in order to keep Mother out of the nursing home." I was shocked, or at least very surprised. Not long after that disclosure, another sister said she wouldn't be helping with the caregiving, and then the "dedicated" one changed her mind.

"If _____ isn't going to help, then I'm not either," she said.

When I asked about her prior commitment to me concerning Mother's welfare and keeping her out of the nursing home, she replied, "But I have to look after *my family.*"

"I thought Mother was part of your family," I answered. "I thought I was part of your family."

"Well, yes, but that's different," she said.

She was now seeing family in a new light or at least telling me for the first time of her feelings. It sounded like a definition of convenience since it only came up when another sister said she wouldn't be helping. "Family" was becoming a cloudy concept to me. Though living across the country, I had still thought of parents, siblings, their children, and in-laws as part of the same big family. During my annual visits home, this thinking was reinforced, and I helped any of the above-mentioned family members whenever they requested it. I admitted to being naïve and was now beginning to realize that the situation had to be faced for what it was. Our mother's welfare was taking a much lower priority than the daily wants of their current spouses and offspring, even if some of them didn't get along well with those spouses.

Before going into the subject further, I want to qualify that this topic is only minimally about my own family. I only use some of our experience as an example to illustrate the condition, to establish some validity, to make the point. More importantly, it represents in whole or in part the condition of countless families across the country. Most importantly, definition of family is an area that should be considered early in life, at least earlier than I did. The health and welfare of all of your loved ones may depend on this. Without some common understanding among all family members, your union can end up like that of fair-weather friends or worse. Many families live with much discord before they are even faced with the extreme challenge of caregiving for an AD patient. However, my siblings and I were not used to having any discord in dealing with each other, so the shock was truly phenomenal.

Several months after my mother passed away, a doctor asked me, "After all the years and experience of caregiving you've had, what one thing would you do differently now if you were starting your care-giving all over?" I said that I would have my siblings, Mother, and me all together to discuss all facets of caregiving, nursing homes and finances. I worked too hard to protect peoples' feelings and absorbed too much of the pain myself. I was a buffer—a liaison between the two elements of parent and the other offspring. Also, I would have the dissenting sisters tell Mother to her face that they wanted to put her in a nursing home. At least I think I would have. Having my siblings be upfront with my mother is what really came to mind. I would be seriously bothered by having my mother face such a painful disclosure even though I would have been there to cushion the blow and remind her of my commit-ment. My mixed feelings on such disclosure relate to the age-old di-lemma of total honesty and candidness which can cause someone great pain, or complete honesty yet partial disclosure in order to spare some-one extreme shock and anguish. To put it another way, it's a matter of being blunt versus being discreet or tactful. Overall, I believe you should be open and honest with your loved one in telling them your intentions. I had no trouble telling Mother of my intentions and commitment. On the other hand, Bernice was a very gentle and sensitive soul who grew even more fragile as her dementia increased, and I wouldn't want to have her exposed to such rejection.

In view of my experience, and with regard to present and future caregivers, I offer the following discussion on the much-used and often-abused term and concept of family.

*****

The term *family* is far more broad-based than most people ever imagine. Similar to the term *love*, it can be defined and qualified in all different types of human interactions. However, for the most part, this word *family* is rarely analyzed by laymen, though in truth it should be.

The concept of *family* is beautiful, but in practice it is often vague and ill-defined. *Family* brings various images to mind. One which we like very much is that of the entire family sitting around the dinner table at Thanksgiving—displaying proper reverence to start the meal and then moving on to the jovial conviviality which everyone desires, a multi-generational blending to share wit and wisdom, a wholesome image, something to strengthen the seams of our familial and social fabric. By questioning this supposedly sacred institution, I may be seen as the grinch who stole Thanksgiving; however, in truth, such advertising images of the cheery turkey-eaters are truly short-lived. They may represent family at its best, but they are not representative of the daily institution.

Christmas may be the ultimate celebration with a family focus for Christians. My parents worked hard to make Christmas a magical time for all of us and to make it a special family event. The gifts were only one part of it and really a lesser part. The spirit of joy and love were much stronger than the material presents. Dad would enjoy reading to us on Christmas Eve the story of the nativity. Those were wonderful times for our family and probably for most other Christian families as well. In fact, the spirit of Christmas permeated society as a whole and joined friends and strangers into a much broader feeling of family, love, and belonging.

*****

In ancient times, family seemed to center around blood relationships. Loyalty was established primarily by blood. Royal sons and daughters from one kingdom were wed to those in another kingdom in order to form pacts and alliances for defense. In later times, the practical application of family involved nepotism—the distribution of jobs and money to blood family members. The expected return was loyalty.

In legal applications, family starts with common blood—grandparents, parents, offspring, uncles, aunts, et al. To begin this chain of events, the conventional first act is marriage. From this union of male and female, we move on to reproduction and children, enlarging the original family of two people.

The definition of marriage is no more a black-and-white issue than is family. While speaking with a friend fifteen years ago, the subject of marriage came up. She said, "The institution of marriage was created for the accumulation of wealth." I don't remember pursuing the subject

further that night, and I don't know which culture or tradition she ac-
quired that information from; however, the words stuck in my mind.
The familial purpose of wealth accumulation may be accurate in many
cases—families striving to build mini-dynasties (e.g., the Rockefellers or
Kennedys). I imagine tribal control preceded marriage, or at least in
terms of to whom we owed our first allegiance and work dividends.

Anyway, soon after children are born, their parents begin to
nourish them and build the children's sense of security, giving them an
identity as new family members. Concerning the children themselves, I
once read that people ask themselves three questions early in life: Where
did I come from? Where am I going? How much time do I have left?
One variation on this probe for understanding is: Where did I come
from? Where am I going? What group do I belong to? Well, the question of which group one belongs to is just another way of asking: Which
family do I belong to? Again, starting at home, we think first of our family as parents and siblings. Then our exposure and training lead us to
other potential "ID badges." There are the matters of race, religion, eth-
nicity, age, culture, geographic designations, sex, mental and physical
definitions, veteran's status, occupations, and of course I should add
caregivers—every one of those categories a possible family designator.
There are so many additional dividers that we can use to separate ourselves from the vast majority of other human beings. As a side note, the
more we define ourselves by these titles or subdivisions, the farther we
get away from the mass of humanity. As an extreme example, if I were
to define myself as a paralyzed, asexual, Hindu male with Attention
Deficit Disorder from South Korea, I would be putting myself in a very
small family, probably a family of one. This last example is quite a
stretch, but I believe that you'll get my point. If I simply define myself as
a human being, then I am in a family of billions and billions.

Families in Conflict

Now, to come back to a more pertinent definition of *family*, I am
reminded of the American Civil War. In this matter, the whole country
was a metaphor for a family in conflict. As President Lincoln said, "A
house [or family] divided cannot stand." In descriptions of that war, I
once read "It was so horrible that sometimes brother was fighting

brother." In another account, the writer stated that the phenomenon of brother-against-brother fighting was so common that the Civil War was often called the Brothers' War. Now, that is sibling conflict acted out with extreme violence. To me, this illustrates the different opinions and values that exist amongst siblings—members of the same blood family. These are often unspoken and perhaps unconscious beliefs, but under the right circumstances they come to light and demand attention. I suppose we could even go back and draw on Cain and Abel, or the later division between Isaac and Ishmael that split the Semitic tribes into Jews and Arabs.

A couple of years ago I experienced a perfect example to illustrate such differences. A lady in my class was giving me her name and address and other info we needed for records. I mentioned the uncommon spelling of her common last name, and she offered the following.

"Just before the Civil War, my husband's family lived in Kentucky. As the slavery issue heated up, his great-grandfather—a young man at that time—was very much opposed to slavery and let it be known. After arguing with his family about slavery and his family having slaves, he decided to leave his parents' sizeable estate, move to Indiana, and give up his inheritance. Also, he changed the spelling of his last name and disassociated from the rest of the family." That was, of course, a serious decision about family—permanently detaching from one's blood family, giving up a considerable inheritance, moving to a state whose values were closer to his own, and changing the spelling of his last name. As a postscript—one generation after that incident—one of his Kentucky relatives moved to Indiana and went to look up the family of the man who had moved here previously. When they met, their talk found them as different as their parents had been, and they never had any further contact.

The issue of religion can be another factor of division or cohesion within a family. What if a family member joins a religion which believes that they have the only ticket to Heaven—a variation on the earlier concept of God's favored people? That person has redefined his or her family connection whether openly declared or not. His/her new authority figures are the leaders of the new religion. They hold that person's ticket to Heaven. If the novitiate is a zealot, then he or she believes that anyone—including blood family—is doomed for not being in the

new religion. He or she may continue to take the blood family benefits—for example, security, affection, daily material benefits, and inheritance—and yet consider himself or herself primarily as being a member
of the new church family. That person wants to have things both ways
and doesn't really sacrifice anything, or stand on principle. Accordingly,
such a person may not feel obligated to help with parental caregiving in
the blood family.

Confronting the caregiving experience is a major issue in life.
When family members are faced with it, the matter is not something you
can just stay silent about concerning your own opinions. You could do
better at keeping your choices of religion and politics quiet than the
other matters (i.e., war and caregiving) which require immediate action,
or inaction as the choice may be. In some matters, a person has to
choose and let the choice be known. For our purpose here, the important thing is to take a long-term view. We need to see beyond personal
beliefs on the rights and wrongs of caregiving. More importantly, we
need to realize that making these major decisions defines which camp or
family we will be in long-term.

One final example of family designation revolves around trust. I
think in my own case of several close friendships I developed in childhood and have continued to this day. After I had known one friend for a
few years, he was introducing me to one of his close, trusted blood relatives. He simply told her, "This is Heydon. He's family." All was clear in
an instant, and there were no questions asked. I've had a couple of other
similar experiences. Such an intro is very warming and rewarding. Those
introductions carry great sincerity and make one feel truly part of a family.

*****

Aside from the personal beliefs that individual family members
have, there is also a power structure within the family unit. In olden
days, that may have been the king or tribal chief or clan chieftain. In
contemporary life, the power roles are generally those of mother and
father. These are the authority figures who command attention. They
construct the basic family philosophy, and they also hold the power of
punishment and reward. They also provide instruction and examples of
dos and don'ts. However, regardless of how good a job the parents do
in teaching, each offspring has his or her own inherent nature and is also
subject to outside influences—anything from daily work or school com-

panions to spouses. Still, as a living symbol, parents usually retain some respect and are revered long after their offspring are married and having children of their own. While the parents live, order may be maintained. This can be due to respect or some sort of fear, to include a fear of losing support, or an inheritance if that is involved.

When the parents die, or become mentally disabled and considered by some to be dead, another force can come into play. This could be called a bid for power—an attempt to take the reins from the fallen authority figures. This bid for power happens in many social and political institutions, and certainly the family is no exception. Although we have come to accept power ploys in the larger institutions, when it hits home—the blood family, that is—the matter is no longer so easily accepted. (To illustrate this progression of the decline of family leadership and authority, I used a train as a metaphor and developed a chart which can see seen at the end of this chapter.)

Parents may hope that their offspring retain the good portion of their teachings, but once they are out of the nest anything can happen. Part of that outside exposure will come from random encounters with society, and another part will come from the influence or control of the partners their offspring choose.

As I ponder this rule of order, the classic novel *Lord of the Flies*[1] comes to mind. For those who don't know the story, it is a tale of a planeload of young English male students whose plane crashes on a remote and uninhabited island. The time frame is vague, but the implication seems to be that they're escaping a catastrophic war; in that context, the plane could today represent a rocket full of people launched when our planet is on the brink of destruction. Anyway, all survive the crash and begin to take stock of the situation. While they start out maintaining their accustomed sense of order, it doesn't take long before the structure begins to unravel. In the absence of their standard authority, one can see a raw savagery begin to develop within a portion of the group. They become two separate groups—one represents the order of law, and the other is a reversion to might-makes-right. Ordered discussion of issues diminishes, and brute force takes over. This in turn develops into a blood lust as a boy from the civilized group is killed, principally for disagreeing with the "hunter's group." The established order of law falls victim to a violent, but somewhat ordered, chaos. The two factions of civilized vs. uncivilized behavior are at odds. When authority figures are lost from a family, the potential for this savagery also comes into play. Repressed feelings may come to surface in order to fuel the attacks. The point is that anything can happen.

With reference to the role of established order in our daily lives, consider the dynamic between the police and regular citizens. The police are society's representatives of authority. What if there were suddenly no police? How long would standard law and order survive? How long would it take the law of the jungle to surface? The most effective role the police play in society is in maintaining a presence, acting as a deterrent to lawless groups and individuals who are just waiting to make a bid for power.

I hate to bring it up, but the veneer of civilized behavior is pretty thin, and the parallel to family cohesiveness is closer than most people would like to think. Within hours after the September 11, 2001, (9/11) attack, many gas station owners raised their prices substantially. Here in Indianapolis, a couple gas stations *tripled* their price per gallon. They were later charged with gouging, but the general effect of vulnerability was felt by all people trying to buy gas then. Our neighbor went down to the corner station to get some gas, and witnessed people beeping their horns and nearly coming to blows over who was at the pump first—not a good sign. A week before 9/11, people were enjoying Labor Day barbeques; then suddenly some were at each others' throat. So, family and social ties may be shallower than we'd like to believe.

*****

My hope is that more people will be able to work out such issues as parental caregiving when these serious moments arise affecting the continuity of a family. People can possibly save themselves a great deal of bickering, grief, and legal intervention if they understand the seriousness of the outcome. You think it won't be your family, but statistics bear out the great numbers. I would never in a million years have considered the possibility of conflict with any of my siblings—especially at such a serious time—but it happened. My father considered me naïve in not accepting this possibility, and he was right.

There comes a time when the most serious issues face a family, and choices have to be made. At that point, you can truly find out where people stand. Most important of all, be true to yourself; you're the one you have to face in the mirror each morning. Again, this discourse on family is not about my blood family any more than millions and millions of others who have come face-to-face with this most serious issue of caregiving for a loved one with AD or some other totally disabling illness. This writing is about preparing oneself for a possibly radical change of reality—one that can change one's concept of family forever. As the Boy Scouts say, "Be prepared." Think it can't happen to you? Think again.

In the end, perhaps the best definition of *family* could be found by following the logic of Forrest Gump's "Mama." I imagine she would eliminate any discussion to try and dissect what constitutes a family or why people choose to avoid or accept parental caregiving. She would probably cut it down to five words by saying, "Family is as family does."

Family Caregiving in Alzheimer's Disease

Why is it such a difficult challenge to get sibling assistance in caregiving for a parent disabled with Alzheimer's disease? It would appear as more of a sacred responsibility. Beloved, widowed parent—the person who brought you into this world, who has perhaps done more for you than anyone else, and who now finds herself or himself in need of help and support in handling their crippling and terminal disability.

The challenge is that it is very difficult to get help in caregiving for someone with an illness of unknown length. Further, when that patient has lost his or her memory, some people consider any responsibility to that person as over. Strange? Yes. However, family dynamics can be very strange when they are put to the most difficult tests.

I've heard that some offspring won't help a parent with dementia because they can't accept that the parent doesn't know who the offspring are anymore. Some people also give that reason for not visiting a demented parent or friend in the nursing home. To me, that is a very weak, selfish, and feeble excuse. When a person has truly loved and nurtured you and helped you in so many ways, how can you simply abandon him or her? It's just beyond my comprehension. If I were a person who thought and felt that way, I would also be in a perpetual quandary as to why we bother living at all. People who view the Alzheimer's patient as a zombie of old blood and bones are people who have no soul. Those are people who maintain a shallow existence and may believe that love is just a Hollywood prop.

Other people won't help or visit a demented parent or friend because they are afraid of aging and death. They may fear that somehow the patient's condition will rub off on them. For some reason, the prototype of such a group comes to mind as an elderly person who has had many facelifts, and his or her skin is stretched to the point of splitting. Of course that is only a blatant example. In reality, there are many people of all ages and both sexes who are terribly afraid of aging and death. Alzheimer's disease, aging, and death could be seen as the trinity of denial. Nobody really wants to die, but it's simply part of the overall package. The sooner one comes to grips with that fact, the healthier he or she will be. And, in demonstrating a healthy, working acceptance of aging and death, we have a chance to be a good influence on others. That reminds me of a conversation I overheard between two friends. The first man asked his friend, "What it be?" The second calmly answered, "What is, is." That answer was the best summation I ever heard on the matters of reality and acceptance.

With reference to Mr. Tolstoy's opening comment on happy and unhappy families, I should add that a formerly happy family, when exposed to the most extreme stress, can soon devolve into a very unhappy family. Happy and unhappy definitions are not really so easily defined. There seems to be a lot of gray area in this spectrum; for example, happiness being contingent on certain conditions being met.

Before going further, I should declare that how a family faces and manages this caregiving will be critically important for the future of the patient, other family members, their extended families, the family as a whole, the community, and the entire nation. This is one of those challenges with very far-reaching consequences; for as families are nourished—or not—so goes the true health of the nation.

*****

This matter of family resolution is most timely as Alzheimer's disease is widespread, and the incidence is growing rapidly. The projected number of AD patients for the year 2050 is sixteen million. However, those numbers only represent the patients themselves. The actual number of victims will be several times that figure. Many families will begin to dissipate under the stress of dealing with the disease. Probably no person in the country will remain unaffected. This could potentially change our society for the worse in ways and on a scale most people can't begin to comprehend now.

A recent article in the N.Y. Times[2] referenced the minimal therapeutic value of current Alzheimer's medications. So, there's no indication that drugs are going to handle the problem for us. While medications would be helpful as an adjunct to caregiving for our AD patient, they couldn't be a total solution. Our hearts and souls are quite helpful tools and are really put to the test in this matter. Empathy and love are the most important resources in helping an AD patient through the terminal struggle.

The actions of family members in providing or withholding caregiving for a disabled and dying parent are a very complex matter. The list of reasons for this is lengthy.

First, let's start with the bottom line. I have read the summation of professionals who state that it is most difficult to get caregiving help for patients who have a debilitating illness of *indeterminate* length. So, if you have a family member who is going to die from cancer within six months, you have a better chance of getting help in caregiving from your siblings than if the patient has AD which has a mortality range of two to twenty years after diagnosis. Sad to say, I believe some offspring feel less accountable to their disabled parent when the parent has lost cognitive skills and can no longer recognize those offspring.

Further, I've read that caregiving responsibilities can be worked out within a family unless there is a prevailing mental or emotional illness in the family. However, in the same publication I read that the primary caregiver ends up doing the caregiving alone in half the cases; that is, the primary caregiver also becomes a solitary caregiver. If caregiving responsibilities can be shared except in a dysfunctional family, and half of the families end up with only a solitary caregiver, then the deduction is that the majority of families are dysfunctional. While deductive logic can be faulty in absolutes, it can still provide a pattern. In subsequent readings, as well as personal experience and interviews with other caregivers, I found the premise that caregiving ends up on the shoulders of one person is the most accurate.

When I found myself alone in caregiving, and then involved in some sibling conflict, I knew something was very wrong in the whole process—not simply unjust, but matters going on under the surface which I didn't understand. I also questioned myself and my approach. By expecting help with the caregiving, was I out of line? I couldn't imagine that to be the case. The whole thing was very confusing. It took a lot of thinking, reading, and talking with other AD caregivers to learn more about what was happening to me. I should add that a great deal of personal, emotional pain was present during the whole sibling experience.

I don't want to dwell on my family's experience—nor any other single family's experience—other than to illustrate a point. What's most important here is the matter of families sharing caregiving responsibilities when their loved ones are in such need. By a discussion here, I'm hoping that it will primarily help caregivers who are currently "in the trenches" or who soon will be. Also, I'm thinking of the family members who aren't participating in the caregiving, but want to retain some semblance of a cohesive family during the caregiving and/or after the patient has passed away.

Finally, if other family members don't want to help the primary caregiver, they should just speak out honestly and say so—even that is better than making some contrived complaint to avoid expressing one's true feelings. The primary caregiver needs to know where he or she stands with regard to supplemental help so that an effective caregiving plan can be developed for the AD patient. One of my siblings was very upfront about not helping with the caregiving, and I appreciated the honesty, even though I was disappointed with her choice.

*****

The stress and loneliness of the primary—and often solitary—caregiver for an AD patient are difficult to describe. Recently, I saw AD caregiving appropriately described as a health risk, similar to cigarettes and excessive drinking. When you add that stress to the additional stress from family members who complain but never help, then you are speaking of serious health risks for the caregiver. It may not be as intense as going into a free-fire zone in combat, but in the long run it can take just as much out of a caregiver—the longer the caregiving, the more costly the toll on the caregiver's health.

I have known, and read of, so many caregivers who were left alone to do the caregiving. There has been a great deal of anger and bitterness, demonstrated as well as hidden. There are caregivers who wouldn't, and haven't, talked with their non-helping siblings for many years, if ever. One thing I knew for sure was that I didn't want to be one of those embittered primary caregivers left with a festering wound. I completely empathize with those caregiver feelings, but holding onto them can be crippling and a way to defuse them must be found. I cover this in the next chapter which is about forgiveness.

With AD patient numbers growing at an incredible rate, such cases could expand to many millions. Imagine what that will do to the social fabric of our country—families disintegrating and subsequent off-spring becoming even colder and more emotionally hostile. When the next generation finds their parents need such care, they may decide to just drop them by the side of the road as some callous and cold-hearted people now do with pets they have decided to abandon. As ye sow, so shall ye reap, if not worse.

While interviewing many AD caregivers, I heard that story again and again and again—primary, solitary caregivers left with the full re-sponsibilities of caregiving for their loved one. Though I seldom heard caregivers truly complain of the task itself, it is so easy to detect the stress and tiredness in their voices. Even though such caregiving is most often done as a labor of love, it still takes a serious toll on the caregiver.

My assumption was that with five children here, we would be able to share my mother's care. I would take the larger share since I was close at hand. In retrospect, I can see that I was naïve about believing that we would all be involved in her care. During my annual vacation trip, I would make sure to get together with my sisters at least once—but usually more—during those visits. It was always upbeat, fun and festive. Perhaps most important, I felt that we were very united.

A year before his death, and while I was home, my father and I were having a conversation one night. He said that I better put my name on the furniture pieces I wanted. Further, the girls had already taken some home, so it was important to label what I wanted.

My parents had a lot of antiques. Some were family pieces that they had had forever. Others were pieces they had bought at auctions mainly in the '60s and '70s, and then Dad had refinished them. He did some beautiful work, and it was a good tool for relieving some of his frustrations and manic energy. When Dad said I should label those I wanted, I replied, "Dad, my sisters and I would never argue over such things. We wouldn't have that kind of problem."

Very calmly, with the air of a person who knows exactly what he's talking about, he said, "Oh yes, you will. I've seen it a million times." It was a little unsettling to hear his reply—not because of the content but because of the manner in which he said it. I should have noted his abnormal calmness which, though rarely seen, always proved that he was on target. Still, he was only completely right about one sibling; however, one is all that it takes if that person is very unhappy, looking to blame someone else, and has a lot of time on his or her hands.

Anger at Family Abandonment

When I found myself alone in caregiving and at odds with some of my siblings, I thought, "What's going on here?" It wasn't really anger that first came to me but confusion. How could a family who had been so close for so many years now suddenly be in such conflict? Was I saying something wrong? Were there dynamics that I just didn't know about? Why wouldn't people help? Is guilt causing them to react badly? As it turned out, the reasons were individual and personal for each sibling. While I considered these issues, a strange thing happened. By chance I ran into an older couple who worked nearby, and who had been friends of my parents for many years. They were very interested in Mother's welfare and asked how things were going. "Pretty good," I replied. "Mother and I get along great, and we're getting organized for different tasks. I am having some problems getting help from my sisters, and that's a puzzle."

Elizabeth looked with a knowing smile toward her husband and said, "I can see it already. He's going to end up like I did." Then she went on to tell me that with all her brothers and sisters no one would help her care for her parents in their infirmities and descent. She spoke with some bitterness that still lingered years and years after her parents had passed away. She still wasn't speaking with any of her siblings.

Following the second parent's funeral, one of Elizabeth's sisters approached her to ask for Elizabeth's help. She told Elizabeth that another of their sisters had kidney disease and may need a transplant to survive. Elizabeth was the only match who would be a suitable donor.

After thinking about it for a while, Elizabeth replied, "You can tell her that I'll give her a kidney, but I won't talk to her."

Needless to say, those are pretty strong feelings. Anger, bitterness, personal hurt, and a sense of betrayal were deeply embedded in her memory. Yet love also remained. I don't know if they normally played any part in her daily life; however, they were close enough to the surface that mention of my situation brought them to the forefront very quickly.

Elizabeth was also in charge of her parents' estate. I don't believe they had made out a will. After debts were paid off, it was a very small estate, but her siblings were anxious to get what they considered their due. That left another portion of bitterness for Elizabeth. I can understand some of Elizabeth's feelings. Why would people who abandon their parents and contribute nothing toward caregiving, who don't support the caregiver and are in fact hostile, still expect to receive a portion of their parents' remaining estate? As a matter of conscience, it just seems strange.

To me, inheritance money is a strange issue anyway. I can see it as a windfall, like winning a portion of a lottery. However, I don't believe that anyone really earns or deserves a financial inheritance. Worse yet, numerous offspring believe their parents' money belong to the adult children already, even while that parent is still living and at home. As a result of that thinking, many elderly have been forced into nursing homes prematurely. Now, the Council on Aging screens potential nursing home residents to make sure they aren't just being dumped in nursing homes for someone's convenience.

My mother's estate was small before she went into the last nursing home. Half of that money had been set aside in a trust for the five offspring years before. If needed, that money could be used for her benefit later. The other half of Mother's estate was used for the costs of nursing homes, and for some professional health aides who supplemented my caregiving at home during the last eight months Mother was able to stay at home. I would take a twelve-hour shift, and the hired aide would take the second twelve-hour shift. The aides were a big help since I could not do it alone at that point.

Mother's doctor had ordered twenty-four-hour care at that stage, and without the aide's help I would have had to put her in a nursing home that much earlier. The extra eight months at home, and subsequent increased dementia, made it possible for her to not realize she had to stay in the facility when I took her. I was grateful to God for that. To realize she was being permanently put in a nursing home would have really broken her heart and, subsequently, mine. She knew she was in a convalescent center but couldn't quite put it all together.

When Mother had been in the nursing home for two years and all her financial affairs were settled, we five offspring received the money from the trust mentioned earlier. Since I still considered that to be Mother's money, I tried to figure out how to best use my portion of it for her benefit.

After Mother went to the nursing home, I had taken a job as a technical writer with a very long work schedule, leaving little time for visiting during my nightly trips to the nursing home. I decided to leave that job and use the windfall money to buy extra time for monitoring operations at the nursing home. There seemed to be some poetic justice in this—a chance to give her the real benefit of the trust money. (I'll speak more about that period in the chapter on nursing homes.)

Solitary Caregivers

A few months after my conversation with Elizabeth—the first primary/solitary caregiver I mentioned—Mother had a TIA and had to go to the hospital for a few days. Then her doctor required she be sent to a convalescent center. I was notified that I had three days to find a nursing home before she had to leave the hospital. That was a shock— to learn that she had to go to a nursing home, and that there were only three days to find one that was decent, met her medical needs, and had an open bed.

I finally found a nursing home and got her situated. Soon after, I went to a care plan meeting where various staff members made recommendations for her care. The Director of Nursing (DON) asked if any of my siblings would be coming to the meeting.

"No," I replied, "I'm the only one involved in her care."

She looked at me understandingly and said, "Oh, you too, eh?"

"What does that mean?" I asked.

The DON then replied, "When it came time for the caregiving, did you suddenly find that you were an orphan also?"

Then she and I spoke for a while about each being the only one from a group of offspring who did the caregiving. The similarities were just incredible. I told her I was surprised to be meeting other people that had happened to.

"Don't be surprised," she answered. "There are a lot of us out there."

The year after that I decided to do some research on family conflict in parental caregiving. I went to the medical section of the main library and requested an index, then a series of published research studies in gerontology journals on family conflict in caregiving. The research librarian gathered the publications and then brought them out to me. She was curious about my interest in that specific topic. After I told her, she said, "I know that situation so well." She had also been left alone with the caregiving responsibilities, and it had marked her deeply.

More recently, I went to a clinic to view Mother's past medical records and told the nurse my purpose in securing the technical info. She said she felt another book on caregiving would be helpful. Then she went on to tell me how she had been abandoned by her siblings to the parental caregiving. I couldn't believe how many people this happened to. I had to assume that these past and present caregivers were keeping that info in the closet until they accidentally found someone in the same boat. Then they really had a need to talk about it. How many people are living with this burning secret of latent anger or bitterness?

Concerning my own case, I felt the same anger and sense of betrayal as so many other caregivers. The pain and anger of dealing with sibling antagonism were just overwhelming. I had to find some answers and a solution in order to continue effective caregiving and to maintain some true mental and emotional well-being. Otherwise, I would be locked in my anger and of diminished help to Mother and myself.

There were several issues and areas I had to figure out. First was the matter of why adult children do or don't help their disabled parents. Second was the issue of what constitutes a family. Third was the matter of dealing with my feelings. Finally, I had to confront the issue of forgiveness if I were to live an effective and satisfying life. Again, I offer my thoughts and experiences in the hope that they may be of help to others who may face—or, are currently living—this painful situation.

Choosing Parental Caregiving, or Not

The choice of adult children concerning caregiving for a disabled and dying parent can be a very complex matter. That choice involves the relationship of each offspring to the disabled parent, and the relationship of each child to their other siblings. Also, there is the matter of what personal problems the offspring may have, and how serious those problems may be. Further, there is the issue of the adult child's extended family—that is, spouse and children—and what influence that family has over their decision.

Family dynamics are never more thoroughly tested than in this situation. At the death—or full mental disability—of the final parent, and subsequent death of the original household, the family structure is strongly tested; but that is for a shorter period of time; that is, division of property, choosing family furniture, etc.

I will try not to enter my personal experience here except as it might be used in a subjective way. I will say that my family went through disagreements which I never would have imagined possible. Ultimately, that just meant that we were regular people who fell into the normal trap.

From what I've read, some of the most common reasons that siblings give for not helping the caregiver are:

1) **Favoritism**—"She/He always liked you more than me…" This one was not an issue in our case. One of my sisters made a point at Mother's Memorial of saying how fair Mother was with all of us.

2) **Long Distance**—"I live too far away to help…" This also was not a problem in our case since I had moved back to Indianapolis in order to be a caregiver. (In self-evaluation, I imagine that if I had stayed in California I could have been a phone nuisance checking to see that everything was being done for Mother.)

The issue of long distance caregiving has recently taken on a new twist. Instead of offspring having moved away, there are many retirees who have moved to warmer climates and eventually disabilities set in. The retirees don't want to leave their warm climate so offspring try to deal with that situation by long distance.

3) **Time**—"I just don't have time to help..." I did hear this one from a sibling. So, I shared some info with her. "Here's how time works. All humans have twenty-four hours in a day. In other words, we all have the same amount of time. It's just a matter of how you're going to divide it. What you mean to say is that you have other priorities for your time. That's okay, but just tell it like it is."

Consider how often in everyday life we hear and use this term—"I don't have time." It seems to be more of a non-answer or brush-off reply. When used as a reply, "I don't have time" usually translates to "I'm not going to do it. I have other priorities. Don't ask me any further."

4) **Training/Patience**—"I don't have the skills or patience to be a caregiver..." There can be other variations on this. For example, there are people who don't want to be around the aged or elderly. If that's the case and they can't get over it, then there are plenty of other things they could do to help the caregiver and AD patient.

Those are some of the common reasons/excuses for not helping the caregiver. When it comes to private reasons for not helping, there can be deeper issues on a list that could go on and on and on. For example:

- Unresolved or unrealized sibling conflict that lay dormant in at least one sibling's mind.
- Sibling with agoraphobia and other personal problems.
- Siblings compromised by alcohol or other drugs. (Would you want them to be caregiving for your loved one anyway?)
- Siblings who simply hate their parents.
- Siblings with untreated mental or emotional illness.

Those are just a few other reasons, but it demonstrates a wide range of possibilities.

The above list of reasons deals with the immediate family members themselves. What about the spouses of those family members? What if spouses control what your siblings will or won't do to help? For example:

- A spouse who didn't like his in-laws and doesn't want his wife to help with caregiving.
- A spouse who doesn't want his wife to serve anyone but him.
- A spouse who had bad parental memories from childhood and takes it out on his or her in-laws, resulting in not allowing his wife/her husband to help the needy parents.

Again, these are just a few of countless reasons or excuses that people will, or won't, give for not helping in parental caregiving. The reasons encountered for not helping in caregiving may be as individual as the individual cases of AD themselves. The dismal point to realize about such family crisis situations is that the norm is to have conflict, often serious conflict. From what I've read, it's very common for formerly happy and healthy families to fall into this trap.

Basically, this issue of having to face parental caregiving on such a widespread scale is new. In old times, there were no nursing homes, and many relatives took care of each other. Also, people died at a younger age and worked until death or close to it. Now we have extended life through pills and procedures—an extension of the 20th century adage "Better living through chemistry." We see films promoting the glory of scientific discoveries all the time, some of it propaganda from pharmaceutical companies. This is not to say there aren't some very good medical discoveries being made. However, there is the matter of whether or not most people can afford them. Currently, a topic of concern among seniors is whether they should use their money to buy medicine or food. Already, a number of Americans are traveling out of country to buy their medicines at a considerably lower price in Canada.

Even then, this new extended life begs the larger question— does this mean a longer life of poverty, abandonment by your offspring when you are in need, and an extended existence of neglected, sub-life in an understaffed nursing home? I don't believe most of us would choose that, at least most baby boomers and younger people wouldn't. Science can begin to replicate the structure of hormones and other chemical processes in our bodies, but they can't construct empathy and compassion for the human heart.

A few years ago I heard a good line from a songwriter and musician who closed his show by yelling to the crowd, "Remember, in the end, nobody wins unless everybody wins!" Incorporating that thought with the action of "Do unto others as you would have them do unto you" could help people rediscover their own souls, and how they relate not only to their immediate blood family but far beyond to the entire family of man.

The final major consideration in dealing with parental caregiving is the matter of guilt. If you have a beloved, respected parent—or perhaps most any parent—who needs your help, and you choose not to help for whatever reason, you will probably face an uneasiness resulting in a sense of personal guilt. If it doesn't happen to you right away, it could well happen later on, even up to the time of your death.

My decision to become a caregiver for Mother was based on several reasons, including the fact that I truly could not have lived with myself if I hadn't taken the stand that I did. She was not only my parent and Mother, but a phenomenal human being and a person whom I loved very much. To abandon her would have been the equivalent of saying that life is meaningless; that we don't owe anything to anyone for any reason. That would be a world without any soul.

Speaking with other caregivers, I found their feelings weren't that much different from mine. They could see how they'd feel down the road if they hadn't chosen to help. That wasn't the motivation for my decision to be a caregiver, but in later thought I realized it—that nothing could be more pitiful than a deathbed regret of not having done the right thing for someone who had done so much for me and so many other people.

For those who believe they should help their loved one but don't do it, guilt can also result in immediate action. It can result in their taking legal action—a petition for guardianship. That takes family conflict to a new level. With guardianship, one has full control over another person's life. One can force the senior into a nursing home, regardless of how the old person feels about it. One can alleviate or dismiss any feelings of guilt in not helping the parent by simply forcing him or her into a nursing home—out of sight, out of mind, much less uneasiness. The matter of guardianship is also a lucrative area for certain lawyers whose incomes thrive on such family disagreements.

Matter of fact, one of the admission requirements for entry into a nursing home is a screening by someone from the Council on Aging, as mentioned previously. The reason for this is that too often people are trying to force their elderly parents into nursing homes when they don't need a nursing home; it is for the relative's convenience, or some financial gain. The government wants to stop this, probably because they often have to foot the bill and not because of the rights of the elderly themselves.

Shock—Petition for Guardianship

This was the worst of the sibling stings. I had originally placed this recounting in the nursing home section where it fell chronologically. However, on second thought, it seemed more appropriate in the family chapter, so I've included it here.

After Mother had been in NH #1 for nearly three weeks, I received the biggest shock of my life. I had a postal notice that there was a registered letter for me at the post office. After signing for it at the post office and reading it, I learned that one of my sisters had filed for guardianship. Driving home with that guardianship notice in hand, I was truly in shock. Having worked to keep my life simple and free of lawyers and legal matters, I didn't really understand what guardianship entailed; however, I knew that it was serious.

That day I was meeting with the owner of a home health agency concerning Mother's needs at home. We were formalizing the home care plan. Since he had years of experience in elder care, I wanted his opinion on this legal notice. Still in shock, I showed him the court paper and asked, "What does this mean?"

He replied very evenly, "This means you're at war." He went on to say that guardianship meant taking complete control of a person's life—the patient would have no say in their destiny, and the Health Care Representative would be overridden, and all health decisions would be made by the guardian.

Further, he added that if I were going to contest this action, I would have to hire a lawyer. Hiring a lawyer would be a very expensive drain on my personal assets—the resources I needed to continue as Mother's caregiver and as her designated Health Care Representative.

My shock was quickly being joined by incredible hurt, anger, and a horrible sense of betrayal. How could my sister do this to me, and to

Mother? And it was done without any warning whatsoever. Was this really happening?

Later, to my true horror, I found out that the filing for guardianship had been agreed upon by three of my four sisters. They had also lured my oldest sister into the lawyer's office on the pretense of concern about Mother's welfare; however, when she saw that the others had a private agenda, she quickly opted out of that cartel. When I later saw one of the trio bringing the court action at the nursing home, I asked her, "Why did you do this? How could you do this?" She replied with a smile and an effort to downplay the matter by saying, "Oh, Heydon, that guardianship hearing doesn't mean anything. It's just a formality, paperwork." Obviously, she wanted me to just forget about the petition and simply let the petitioner have guardianship.

That wasn't going to happen. I contested the guardianship petition, and they unhappily learned that their request wouldn't be a cut-and-dried court action. The early February hearing was postponed for 45 days until March 22, 1995, due to my contesting the action.

How could this happen to our group of siblings who had been so close for so many years? How could these sisters do this to Mother and me—people who had loved them so much and done anything they ever asked of us? There had been no sign of conflict among us in all our years. As I so painfully tried to piece this puzzle together—that is, how such a thing could happen to our family—I went back over the years of caregiving, as well as years prior to this condition. I remembered Dad's warning.

Anyway, this was the load I was carrying. I had to work through the logistics of Mother's care—at the nursing home and then planning for her return home; I had to try and soothe the emotional pain she continually felt at being in this strange and unfavorable environment; and then, hardest of all, I had to digest and accept this horrible sibling betrayal.

Now I would have to hire a lawyer and probably use my savings—and perhaps retirement account as well—in order to slay the dragon and allow Mother her wish to stay home. Or, I could be risking all that and lose in court with the result being much of my money gone, and Mother forced into a nursing home anyway.

At some point I must have thought, "Why did I leave my simple, pleasant life in California?" However, that wouldn't have been a serious thought, for I was dedicated to helping Mother through this disease. The bottom line was that I was all she had, and she had entrusted her care to me. I had never denied my sisters anything they wanted, but I wouldn't tolerate their forcing Mother into a nursing home before her time. Their not being willing to help with her care was one thing; however, trying to force her into a facility for their own convenience, to alleviate their own guilt, and/or for personal gain, was another matter entirely.

One thing that disturbed one sister, and probably the other two siblings in line with her, was the reality of how much it cost to have professional aides helping Mother for twelve hours a day. However, the doctor had said 24-hour care was necessary, and by that point I could do no more than twelve hours of hands-on caregiving a day by myself. Somehow, my three siblings had managed to forget that it was Mother's money, and since she wanted to stay at home, those outside aides would be necessary. The judge was about to remind them.

Before court date, March 22, 1995, I tried to appeal to my siblings—the three petitioners—to find a solution without going to court. One suggestion I made was that we share the caregiving duties and take it in one day or twenty-four-hour shifts each on a rotating basis. Through that suggestion, we could have avoided the cost of the additional aides and also kept our family out of a public courtroom. I didn't receive any reply to the suggestion. I suppose that wasn't surprising considering they weren't involved in caregiving to begin with.

The night before court I thought about how hard the result would be for Mother if the petitioner were awarded guardianship. That is, the trio would quickly send Mother to a nursing home. Mother would understand what had happened and then truly end up with a broken heart. At that stage, I would be powerless to stop it. I didn't pray for help that night. My prayer was simply, "Thy will be done."

Court Day

We were in court for several hours. It was a long process as each of us was called up to testify and be cross-examined. Mother came to court and answered questions put to her by the judge. She was allowed to keep her seat and not come up to the official testifying seat. She sat with Pat and Nancy, and she seemed pretty cheerful. Also, there was an affidavit from Mother's doctor testifying to her condition, but the content was not what the petitioners had hoped for. The doctor wrote that by Mother's appearance and demeanor, I had been doing a good and conscientious job in her care.

In the end, their court action backfired on them. Since a guardian now *had* to be appointed, the judge felt I would be the best personal guardian. I imagine part of his decision was based on the fact that the three sisters/daughters had not been involved in Mother's care during the last four years—other than the sister who had Power of Attorney (POA) and paid Mother's bills—so they had no track record in caregiving and their motives might be questionable. I, who had never thought of the need for legal guardianship, was suddenly made personal guardian.

Further, the judge called into question some of the financial decisions the POA had made. She, her husband, and the other two sisters supporting her guardianship had all benefited financially from Mother's funds. One sister had received large gifts for her daughter. Another sister had been given very large loans of Mother's money that weren't repaid. Finally, the POA had bought large financial policies from her husband, and they benefited substantially from those. I should mention here that my fourth sister—the one that the others had tried to conscript into their court action but who had refused—had not benefited financially from Mother's funds. I knew about those bad financial choices by the POA, but I wouldn't have brought them to court on the matter. That wouldn't have helped anything.

According to a summary portion of the court transcript, the judge ruled as follows, "This Court thinks that you can't take it with you and if you have money and it is reasonable to spend money to care for someone, even large amounts of money to care for someone in a way they need care, that money ought to be used until it's all gone. It's not the children's money until someone is deceased. It is the person's money for their own care. ...I'm troubled by the making of loans. I'm troubled by the—the sale of insurance products by the power of attorney's husband to the Ward. ...Those things look terrible and they're suspicious...and it shouldn't have happened that way. ...We also, in this court, have a problem with the giving away of money of someone who is incapacitated. She—Bernice Buchanan is not incapacitated just as of this day, even though the judicial finding is made this day. That happened some time in the past. And at the point where that happened, she was no longer able to approve of any kind of loans or gifts; she didn't have the capacity to. And where that's the case, it doesn't matter what she did when she did have capacity. It doesn't matter what the family did, she doesn't have the capacity and the guardian has no authority, the power of attorney has no authority, nobody has any authority after she loses that capacity. ...I'm saying, certainly they look suspicious. If she had no capacity, they're wrong...."*   *Hearing on Petition for Appointment of Guardian, Judge's Comments & Ruling—March 22, 1995 (State of Indiana, Marion County, Marion Superior Court, Probate Division)

So, that was the court report. I'm sure the four people involved, and they were all in the courtroom, were embarrassed about that reprimand and quite unprepared for those financial decisions to be questioned at all. The POA's husband was in the back of the courtroom in dark sunglasses in an already low-light courtroom. He may have had a premonition of what was coming. The judge was completely right in his decision and summary. It hadn't been difficult for the judge to tell what was going on.

Eventually, the court appointed a financial guardian (a local lawyer) for Mother, and I was appointed the personal guardian. The financial guardian paid Mother's bills while I was in charge of Mother's health and daily welfare. The three sisters' actions cost Mother about $15,000 in legal fees when the financial guardian's fees were included. That money was a sizable portion of Mother's holdings, and it was completely wasted by the senseless action of three troubled people. The loans, gifts, and commissions to the four people involved wouldn't be recovered either, so approximately $25,000 to $30,000 of Mother's money was wasted or misused by those people. In fairness to two of those three sisters, I should add that they seemed to drop any antagonism after the court action. The judge made himself clear, and there was nothing left for them to say. The court action had backfired on those women, most visibly on the person who had filed for guardianship.

The court action was a nightmare and unbelievable to me. Yet, my attorney said that such actions are very common. More recently, I reflected on the story of King Lear—the tragedy written by Shakespeare. In that scenario, the dementia patient and his caregiver were taken to court by two of the caregiver's sisters. In our case, the dementia patient and her caregiver were taken to court by three of the caregiver's sisters. Otherwise, all essential details were the same in both cases. Shakespeare wrote that story four hundred years ago, and that illustrates how unchanging human nature can be.

*****

An acquaintance of mine jokingly called those three sisters "the three evil stepsisters," as in the case of Cinderella. But that is not really indicative of their character. I believe they were under the influence of something or someone, and they just weren't thinking right. Many such people become misguided, but I never thought it would happen in my family. In any event, I know Mother would forgive them, and I've forgiven them. So, it's past.

I should add that those sisters are essentially honest people. When Dad was previously in L.A. and told me his choice for POA out of the four sisters, I agreed with him. She was a little more grounded than the others. However, I imagine her weakness in that case as being susceptible to pressure from others. When I had questioned one of those others earlier about some frivolous spending of Mother's money, she replied, "Well, it's up to the POA to decide how to spend the money." That was the sum of her logic. Spending in Mother's interest was not part of that logic. It was becoming like kids at the cookie jar.

One of my sisters told me that the POA and her husband were worried for a long time that I was going to sue them. I suppose I could have, but I can't imagine how suing would help the situation at all. I didn't want to sue, and I'm sure Mother wouldn't want me to. The money that they'd misused and wasted was simply gone. They had just made some bad choices, and the judge straightened them out. It wouldn't serve anyone to prolong such agony.

To emphasize that I still considered Dad's choice for POA as valid, I offer a further example. A year after the court action, and when Mother was permanently placed in the nursing home, I left a letter in Mother's medical record saying that _____ (the former POA) should be chosen as guardian in the event of my death before Mother's. I still considered her Mother's best hope if something should happen to me.

So, Mother and I just continued on with handling the disease and its heartbreaking effects. And, I had the added task of protecting her from knowledge of that negative activity.

*****

Again, my family was not at all unique in having problems with caregiving for an Alzheimer's patient. Our circumstances—just like those of any other family—are simply singular in their personal dynamics. Being faced with parental caregiving choices is akin to having fully-committed, candid discussions of religion and politics—a person's real and true beliefs are put on the table, consequences be what they may.

Most importantly, there have been, and continue to be, millions of other primary, solitary caregivers like myself—people who face serious family disagreements and find themselves almost, if not totally, alone as they endure the pain and anger of being abandoned and abused at this time, while they are also under the heavy stress of caregiving. Hopefully, by putting my sibling experience on the stage, other caregivers who currently suffer may find some understanding and not feel so alone. Also, potential, future caregivers may have some warning about the dire possibilities inherent in the caregiving decision—not to dissuade them from making the caregiving choice but simply to prepare them.

I debated with myself for years and years about whether to write this for distribution. Being such a private person, I didn't want such immaturity to be made public, even if it only reflected badly on them. Also, I thought my parents would be disappointed to see this happen. On the other hand, the matter was already public by the guardianship action which the three brought to a public courtroom. Further, my parents always contributed to community and public service, and that is the purpose of my writing about this now—to help other families in the same boat or to warn others who are about to face this most serious family testing ground. With the rapidly growing number of AD patients and the accompanying issue of parental caregiving, potential victims need as much help as they can get, in and out of court.

I can still hear my father's voice warning me of the sibling problems to come. I was almost arrogant in replying to him that my sisters and I would *never* have such a problem. However, now I have to completely concede to his words of wisdom—you were right, Dad.

*****

In sum, facing the parental caregiving issue has more serious potential for making or breaking a family than any other issue I can think of. It is a time to try and be objective and face all the issues as honestly as possible. Handling death is simple compared to the often serious quandary of long-term parental caregiving. If your family has success-fully made it through this most difficult time—sharing caregiving re-sponsibilities and avoiding hostilities—consider yourself very fortunate, for you are in a real minority. I heard one person say that he and his sib-lings had done it without arguments, etc., and he seemed to be gloating about that. I think that attitude is a mistake. That's like a person saying he's proud that he's physically healthy when he hears that his neighbor got cancer. Whether body, mind or soul; whether you, your neighbor, or a family in Botswana; illness is illness, and we need to contribute what knowledge and experience we've gained in order to try and eradicate it for everyone. What we have to remember in facing this situation is that everyone involved is dealing with a series of difficult emotions—loss, anger, denial, etc. Emotions simmer and flash in this period, and very quickly the cauldron can explode. Try to remember that we are all hu-man and fall short of the Glory of God.

A couple of months ago, I saw a TV program where a wealthy celebrity with an Alzheimer's affected parent was speaking about a movement to save the family memories before the AD patient gets too advanced in dementia to remember. While I believe that's a good idea, I also believe that the first priority should be saving the family itself.

*****

Just recently, while finishing this manuscript, I received a letter from my youngest sister apologizing for her role in the trio's antago-nism. She wrote, "Dear Heydon: ...If at some point, we need to talk about all the insanity, I am willing. But mostly I just want you to know that I realize you did what you thought best and I thank you for it. For my part, I was just emerging from the _____ and _____ fog and not thinking clearly at all. ...I know it was a devastating time for you, and for that I offer my most humble apologies, that I was not more helpful to you. ...Our mother was a dear person. I remember some stellar say-ings from her: 1) always look for the GOOD in others; 2) it's important to know how to untie knots, no matter how snarled; 3) when you're troubled, stay busy; 4) look for treasures (rocks, leaves, flowers); 5) al-ways give the other person the benefit of the doubt; 6) always try to make-do with what you have (i.e., make the best of things). I know there

are more, but these are off the top of my head. They come to me often.
...Love, _____ ."

*****

My relationship with each sibling is different; that is, according
to how far we've strayed from each other during these past fifteen years.
My oldest sister and I never quarreled so that's not a problem. My
youngest sister apologized for her behavior. Another sister is pleasant
and invited me to come by anytime. The fourth and final sister still remains a mystery. While I'm not sure what the future holds for some of
us in terms of personal relationships, perhaps we can meet on a new and
higher level of understanding—a sort of rebirthing. It is notable when a
person recognizes and admits his or her mistakes. It provides hope. Taking such an action is also the first step on the road to a family's recovery,
and we were all in need of recovery, each of us for different reasons.
Healing was definitely on my mind as I wrote the next chapter—the
matter of forgiveness.

FAMILY IN TRANSITION

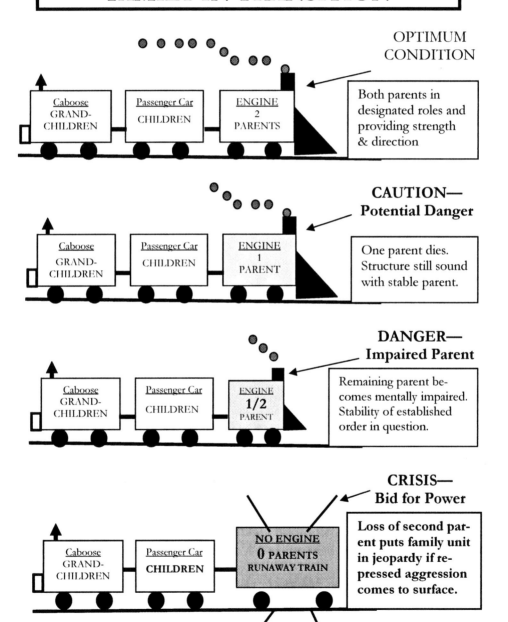

OPTIMUM
CONDITION

Both parents in
designated roles and
providing strength
& direction

CAUTION—
Potential Danger

One parent dies.
Structure still sound
with stable parent.

DANGER—
Impaired Parent

Remaining parent be-
comes mentally impaired.
Stability of established
order in question.

CRISIS—
Bid for Power

Loss of second par-
ent puts family unit
in jeopardy if re-
pressed aggression
comes to surface.

CHAPTER 6

FORGIVENESS

21 Then Peter came and said to him, "Lord, if another
member of the church sins against me, how often should
I forgive? As many as seven times?" 22 Jesus said to him,
"Not seven times, but, I tell you, seventy-seven times."
   —The Gospel of Matthew, Chap. 18, Verses 21-22

Holding on to anger is like grasping a hot coal with the intent of throwing it at someone else; you are the one who
gets burned.
   —Buddha

It is easier to forgive an enemy than to forgive a friend.
   —William Blake

Forgetting is something that time takes care of, but
forgiveness is an act of volition, and only the sufferer
is qualified to make the decision.
   —Simon Wiesanthal

To carry a grudge is like being stung to death by one bee.
   —William H. Walton

THE ISSUE OF FORGIVENESS COMES UP IN CAREGIVING AT LEAST AS
often as it does in everyday life. Forgiveness is called for when one
person has caused another to have some pain or distress. Resolving the
situation often becomes a matter of giving or getting forgiveness, and
then moving on.

     Forgiveness is just one of the trials a caregiver faces during, or
after, the process of caregiving. At times I see the whole journey of

caregiving as a combination of the epic voyage The Odyssey and the more contemporary trip of Pinocchio. The AD caregiver is engaged in a perilous mission. She or he must leave the comfort of the known world and make their way through an unknown and fearful world, passing through a variety of serious obstacles to help their patient more comfortably reach a place of peace. If that mission is successfully accomplished, the caregiver becomes a more complete or realized person and reaches a place of peace as well. Acts of forgiveness are notable milestones on that journey.

In caregiving—with so much intense human interaction—the need for forgiveness can come up quite often. While it need not be consciously considered after every "situation," there are instances where neglecting it will disable a person. If it disables a primary caregiver, the care recipient could be at additional risk. My caregiving experience called for facing the issue of forgiveness in three areas of family involvement. The first area was the care recipient—my mother. The second was the caregiver—myself. The final area concerned other immediate family—my siblings.

*****

I've read that anger—overt or covert—from the caregiver toward the care recipient is very normal behavior. One rationale for that anger is that the caregiver resents giving up her or his life in order to be a caregiver. Another reason is that the caregiver is simply burned out...stressed out...worn out.... Everybody has a breaking point, and when enough of the stressors are in full swing, a person is bound to get angry. Of course how a caregiver releases that anger is the most important point. I was fortunate to find and develop some effective aids to help relieve a lot of stress. I've covered those in an earlier chapter with tools to help the caregiver.

Some caregivers are inherently more patient than others and will be slower to reach the anger point, all other stressors being equal. The caregiver's patience itself may fluctuate according to the depth of love and joy, or negative feelings, which he or she received from the care recipient in earlier life; also, according to how tired, hungry, and stressed the caregiver is at the time.

Concerning anger toward Mother as my care recipient, I don't believe there was any. I've heard this reaction is most uncommon. To me, anger implies blame; that is, when someone or something has consciously or unconsciously done something that hurts you, and you're angry at them. At least, in the rational sense that's the case. In the irrational sense—often possible in AD caregiving—anger is more likely attributed to caregiver general stress overload.

While caregiving for an AD patient can be highly stressful, I never blamed my mother for behavior resulting from her condition. No matter how much pressure I felt during her care, I never blamed her in any way—never thought it, never felt it, never said it. This lady was the kindest and finest person I've ever known, and there was absolutely no way that she would intentionally give another person stress or discomfort. As a result, there was no issue with Mother where I needed to consider forgiveness.

Beyond that, my decision to become her caregiver was a decision of mine alone. She didn't ask me to be her caregiver even though she much appreciated it when I told her it was absolutely my choice. This handles at least the intellectual defense I had against anger. Admittedly, there is another greater factor why anger wasn't a problem in my/our case.

As I remember, Mother didn't act out as is so common with AD victims. She didn't rant or rave or strike out or use profanity or do any anti-social action. That was a big help in alleviating my stress level and subsequent anger from caregiver exhaustion. Mother's principal demonstration of pain was in her anguish, and that was demonstrated by cries and tears. It could be severe during the transitional phases of the disease. Those episodes happened mostly during the last eight months at home when I brought in supplementary caregivers for part of the day. The hired aides gave me a break. At some point, Mother would miss me, not recognize the caregiver, call for me, and then have a crying episode. In referring to my journal, as well as the aides' notes, I see that anguish happened frequently during that period. I've been working to forget the harder times, and after this writing I will try that once again.

It hurt me so much to see her in that pain. I would hold her, and tell her things would be okay; that her pain was part of the disease; and that I would be there for her. Another strategy I had was to distract her, take her mind elsewhere. If she was distressed and in bed for a nap or the night, I would lie next to her and talk to her until she could relax, sometimes giving or promising ice cream as a distraction. Defusing the anguish was always a challenge. It was heartbreaking and extremely stressful to watch someone you love so much have to suffer like that. On the other hand, a few minutes after a heartbreaking episode, she could be laughing at a joke we shared or an old comedy on TV.

Helping an Alzheimer's patient through their difficult and final years can be a very spiritual act, especially in the case of family caregivers who have given up much to take on the caregiving role. The degree of spiritual benefit for all caregivers may be relative to the amount of help given, sacrifices made, and compensation received. For example, professional caregivers (i.e., doctors, nurses, aides) give help to the patient, but they also have a private life. They put in their shift at work and then go home. They receive a paycheck. They have children and spouses and social lives. They have vacations and holidays. They attend school. They advance their careers. They pay off mortgages and build retirement funds for their future. They have ample opportunity to defuse their stress. And, they're not as emotionally tied to their patients as family caregivers are.

On the other hand, family caregivers have often given up everything to take care of their loved ones. Many have given up their up their jobs, seniority, and any hope of advancement. Many have given up their professions since they can't stay current in their field, are soon outdated, and entering the time of age discrimination in employment. They are committed to their loved one's well-being 24/7/365. Many family caregivers are spending their savings and their retirement funds in order to finance their caregiving. So, they're not advancing in their professions and assets, nor are they even holding their own; they are moving steadily downward in many ways, just like their disabled loved ones. However, the family caregiver does have the chance for such spiritual reward as is not available to anyone else. The family caregiver has the chance to understand love and sacrifice as few other vocations, or avocations, can.

*****

I think I flunked at being a normal caregiver if it's normal to have anger toward your care recipient. There may be thoughts of scepticism from some members of the medical community who feel that anger is the norm, but I stand firm on this in my case. That doesn't mean that I wasn't highly stressed and often exhausted by the caregiving experience. And, that doesn't mean I wasn't angered by the actions of others—some in the professional support system and some within our family. I do remember that I had some feeling of relief, among many other feelings, when my care recipient finally had to go in the nursing home, as my abilities were no longer adequate to the task of caregiving at home.

Finally, I should mention that Mother and I have similar natures in being very patient. Patience gives a caregiver a buffer zone before he or she is worn out. Mother could ask me the same question many times in a row, and I would answer it as though it was the first time, and it didn't bother me that she asked the same question time and again. None of the manifestations of the disease were her fault. She was simply the very innocent victim who had to suffer through it internally.

*****

The second case for which to consider forgiveness was for the caregiver himself—me. I tend to be highly self-critical in an attempt to do the right thing. While caregiving for my mother—the person I loved most on earth—that self-critical side of me would be especially active. Questions would often plague me as I reviewed each day: "Did I do this right? Should I have done this instead?" In the midst of high stress, it becomes more difficult to be calm enough to forgive yourself, to simply take it easy on yourself. For me, it was helpful to receive some verbal reinforcement from others about the value and quality of my caregiving. That at least served as a quick fix. When I had a little free time to ponder my caregiving as a whole, I realized how much more I did right than wrong.

Since AD caregiving was new to me—as it must be, or could be, for millions of others in the baby-boom generation—some mistakes were to be expected. Fortunately, none were serious but more a matter of learning how to access other resources to supplement my care. Also, when you are alone as a caregiver, you tend to be more self-questioning. It is truly a lonely position to be a primary and solitary caregiver for an AD patient. Mother's doctor was reassuring during our office visits, but trips to him were few and far between since Mother was otherwise in such good health.

Words of encouragement are especially helpful to the caregiver, and I am reminded of a written example of this comfort. At Christmastime 1992, almost two years into my caregiving, Mother gave each of my siblings, their husbands, her grandchildren, and me some money in an envelope, as shopping for gifts had become too complicated. We all received the same amount. She wrote our names on the outside of each envelope. On the inside she wrote a brief comment to me. Her handwriting, always clear and precise in the past, was now etched with the little stops and starts that illustrate the degeneration of handwriting from the effects of AD. As much a pondering as a comment, she wrote, "Where would I be without you? Much love, Mother." To feel such gratitude from someone who needs you so much in their daily living can provide the caregiver with a lot of fuel for the hard road ahead. Also, to hear it from someone who's done so much for you is very rewarding.

*****

The third and final area for forgiveness during my caregiving experience concerned siblings. This portion is the principal reason for my considering the subject of forgiveness at all. Most people won't write about their experience with siblings at the time of caregiving for elderly and disabled parents. All too often it's an unpleasant experience leaving a bitter taste and something they wish to forget, regardless of whether or not they'll be reuniting with their siblings. Not writing about it is one thing, but not dealing with it is another matter. To not resolve such a major life event can leave a festering wound at some level in the mind and soul. I didn't want to write the chapters about families and forgiveness. Like other primary caregivers in similar situations, I wanted to just forget about that conflict; and for years and years, I wouldn't write about it. In the end, I decided that to not include family and forgiveness would be irresponsible, since those subjects play a major part in AD caregiving for most every caregiver.

By nature, I'm the most private of people. To open up about this sibling disagreement—though some may consider it a light opening—is a radical step for me and painful in itself. However, caregivers need to share their stories so that others facing a similar situation may learn of potential problems. And, caregivers who have been through these family conflicts can hopefully come out of the closet and breathe fresh air, knowing that they are not alone in the conflict they experienced.

I don't think I'm exaggerating when I say the future stability of families in the country is at stake in this matter of AD caregiving—

at least that of the middle class and poor, and these two groups are the foundation of the country. Rich people will simply hire aides and other medical personnel to cover a 24/7 schedule and avoid any of the most serious caregiving stress and family conflict caused by being caught in the vortex of the disease. Otherwise, the lives of the wealthy will not be greatly affected, other than to face the loss of a loved one, and possibly have concerns about familial genetic patterns for inheriting AD.

*****

What family/sibling matters call for forgiveness? I've given some details on this in an earlier section. So, to summarize briefly, primary and solitary caregivers could be angry at not receiving help from siblings in the caregiving and not being appreciated or encouraged in the work. Perhaps worst of all is active hostility toward the caregiver, and this one may result from the personal guilt of not helping with the caregiving. There could be additional resentments toward non-caregiving family members who simply go on with their lives while the caregiver puts her or his life on hold or more likely surrenders it to the indeterminate demands of the disease on his or her loved one and subsequently himself or herself. The primary/solitary caregiver and the unhelpful siblings are living in very different worlds at that point. The circumstances may vary from family to family, but the essence is the same. Since the burden of caregiving appears to fall on one person in at least half of caregiving situations, there can be no doubt about the problems of alienation and the related issues of forgiveness facing so many families. When the caregiver finishes the long road of AD caregiving, she or he may well be depleted of most of their resources—physical, mental, emotional, and financial. At the same time, the non-caregiving siblings and their families may be healthy, financially solid, and approaching retirement. Have no doubt that a wide gulf has been created between the two diverse elements of "the family."

*****

For a number of years, it was very hard to even write this without a mad rush of resentment welling up. The feelings of inconceivable betrayal would rush my mind again and again making clear and ordered thought so difficult. It's impossible for someone who hasn't experienced this to realize the depth of this feeling. To put it in perspective, I would say that receiving a phone call with the announcement that most of your closest loved ones had just died in a plane crash would fall short in comparative pain. That news may be shocking and sorrowful, but it doesn't involve serious betrayal. The pain of the worst betrayal can be horrendous, like a multi-year, mental and emotional crucifixion. I recently read one account of an AD solitary caregiver who couldn't bring herself to speak with her siblings three years after their mother had passed away. Her anger was based solely on not receiving help with caregiving and didn't include the equally serious agitation of hostility and court action. I believe her story to be a common one.

Was there any sense in my holding on to such pain? It would seem not. Relatives who were aware of the problem advised me to forgive. Also, I spoke with a doctor at the VA who wondered why I was holding on to the experience when it hurt so much. That's not a bad question intellectually, but it shows no understanding. Imagine being forced to helplessly watch your family being tortured to death, and afterwards someone says to you, "You've had a bad experience. Now just forget about it." Then, if you didn't quickly do so, someone asks why you want to hold on to that pain. These intense human interactions take time to healthily resolve.

The above example may appear to the uninitiated as foreign and extreme, so I'll offer another scenario. Imagine that your world is turned completely upside down after you have survived an abnormally difficult and stressful situation. Virtually all points of reference are gone, destroyed as you became the repository for someone's misguided hate. We've seen this throughout history on a much larger scale when peoples are dispossessed, tortured, killed, and survivors turned into homeless refugees. It's a horror.

For a long time I tried forgiveness, or at least how I conceived of it. However, the progress of that forgiveness was broken, as one sibling kept needling the situation. Those agitations made it impossible to set the anger aside. It was apparent that she wanted the unhealthiness to continue. The other siblings pretty much settled down, but the instigator—the unhappiest one—continued to agitate. Perhaps I could have considered complete forgiveness even during her actions, but I was too raw and bruised to allow that to pass without mention. More importantly, I found those agitations to interfere with Mother's care, and that care took so much time and concentration that I couldn't tolerate the negative interference. Following the advice of others who were interested in my well-being, I resolved to try and forgive. I've done pretty well with that.

As far as holding on to anger and pain, I've recently thought people may do this unconsciously in an attempt to hold on to a relationship and believe that eventually the offender will come to his or her senses. We keep analyzing the situation over and over, trying to make some kind of sense of it. That is a hopeless struggle. You have to let it go, and you're the only person who can do that.

If I were wiser; if I had had the luxury of time and healing; if I hadn't been facing the minute-to-minute, hour-to-hour, day-to-day stress of Mother's well-being in the battle with Alzheimer's disease, and the challenges of dealing with nursing homes and a myriad of medical personnel; if I hadn't been wrapped up in the concurrent stress of dwindling resources, then I could have focused completely on forgiveness and worked on understanding the various problems my sibling had— problems which probably led her to the unfortunate and negative spot she was in. With enough time and comfort to reflect, I could have understood that her personal situation may have caused her to lash out, to transfer the pain that had been building in her for many years. It's the old story we hear of early in life—the boss yells at his employee; the employee goes home and yells at his wife; the wife yells at their child; the child kicks the family dog; and on.

When a person has time and clarity of mind, she or he can reflect on all these factors and begin to understand. However, when they are active AD home caregivers, they cannot. Time is of the essence, and a million things are going on at once.

To not help with caregiving is one matter; to actively interfere with the caregiving process is another. Once an able-minded person has gone through his or her physician to name a Health Care Representative for when she is no longer able to make her own health care decisions, and when the physician has tested and verified that representative, then the patient's wishes should be respected. Anyone who interferes with an AD patient's health choices after that is a hindrance to the patient's health and well-being.

When I told an old friend about the sibling problem at the beginning, he was truly in shock. Pat and I have been close friends for forty-two years, and he has also been a steady friend of our family for all that time. He was just incredulous and said, "You always held your sisters out there like stars in the sky." There had been absolutely no indication in our sibling history there would ever be a problem.

"I know," I replied. "This is unbelievable."

"When this is all over," he continued, "I can't even begin to imagine the depth of anger you'll have."

Though I had sublimated some of that anger in order to focus on my caregiving, the negative feelings were pretty strong and not healthy for me. That situation would be the principal focus of my work on forgiveness. Again, the anger was not because I didn't receive help with caregiving, but because of the misplaced antagonism of one person and its effect in draining emotional resources that were needed for caregiving. Even that I could have coped with, but their court action took it over the edge. I had never denied my siblings anything they wanted and had often gone out of my way for them. However, as I mentioned earlier, they pushed things over the line when they tried to force Mother into a nursing home. At that point, the easy-going I stepped aside, and the defender came to the surface. After more than forty years, I finally had to say no to those three siblings. I'm sure it was quite unexpected.

*****

Forgiveness is an issue to which we pay lip service from childhood on. Perhaps it started for many of us as children with recitation of the Lord's Prayer, as we settled in for sleep. "...Forgive us our trespasses, as we forgive those who trespass against us...." Then at some point in life we hear, "Forgive and forget" or "Let bygones be bygones."

Why is it so difficult to truly forgive? How many people successfully do it? My guess is that not too many actually "forgive and forget" or even truly forgive.

What I had to realize was how individual the issue of forgiveness really is. The simple jingoisms about forgiveness do not work very well for real forgiveness. As we listen to clergymen, therapists, family and friends who advise us on the issue, there is usually something which doesn't ring true in their textbook advice. It's not that they aren't sincere in offering their counsel; it's that they aren't aware of what it will take each of us individually to recognize that forgiveness into our souls, to have it fully settle into our gut—to move on serenely. True forgiveness is an individual matter and can't be standardized.

*****

First we have to consider what issues even bring on the need to consider forgiveness. Usually, it's after we feel that we've been wronged. The most obvious catalysts are when we feel betrayed, physically or verbally abused, or stolen from. Beyond the various hurts, on a deeper level these perceived assaults seem to threaten our physical survival. And physical survival is the strongest of our basic instincts. The assault may just appear to be a threat to our trust and dignity, but ultimately I believe the unconscious sees it as a threat to our continued existence on earth. For this, our defenses go on full alert.

When we consider giving real forgiveness, we are also considering whether to live our lives beyond common existence—on a spiritual plane that transcends the everyday life of family, work and war. What forgiveness really represents is an opportunity to grow. You may have to leave your pride behind, but which is more important to you—pride or spiritual growth? This may be an appropriate spot for my father's old admonition, "You can't have your cake and eat it too." Or even the wise man saying, "You can't worship God and mammon," for in this case "mammon" represents anything from personal pride to physical existence. So, one can have spiritual growth, or pride and prejudice and the bindings of the ego, but one can't have it both ways.

*****

If you are willing to let go of your pain and anger and resentment, then you are at the starting point. Before you reach that willingness, you are simply lost in your personal suffering. Fueled by rage, you list the trespasses against you and then call for justice. Perhaps justice will come in the form of Karma or "What goes around comes around," but that really won't do you any good. If you witness this "justice," you may feel some satisfaction, or you may even gloat. Seeing this "payback" may help satisfy your sense of revenge, but it does nothing for your growth and true serenity.

So, how do you forgive? How do you pass off the pain of a vast betrayal as though it never happened? First, you might try to realize that there are different views about any situation witnessed by at least two different people. The Japanese film *Rashomon*[1] is an excellent illustration of how three people who saw the same event had very different interpretations. Essentially, we all see things differently. Let's move beyond different interpretations and say that in this situation you are right. Further, there's no question about the facts; you truly have been seriously wronged. However, what's the point of being right if you still feel bad? Justice probably will right a wrong at some point in this life or another, but what matters here and now is your peace of mind. Forgiveness in a family case involves more than just witnessing justice. Beyond justice, there is the breaking of a long-held sacred bond, and that has to be dealt with.

In my case, I finally figured out that forgiveness meant viewing my siblings as human beings instead of highly-trusted members of a close family unit. The unspoken family contract was seriously broken, and that—the most painful of the transgressions—had to be dismissed. It was time for me to stop thinking primarily of family in the traditional sense of close, blood relationships.

*****

So, to sum it up, do what you have to do to forgive. If necessary, dismiss the simple blood connection and cultural training that bind you to your unhappiness. To paraphrase the Nazarene, "Who are my mother and sisters and brothers? Whoever does the will of God is my brother, and sister, and mother."

If members of your primary blood family are positive forces, and you are interested in each other's welfare, that is good. It gives you a base to start from, and can then be supplemented by your new family members at work, in school, the military, marriage and offspring, fraternal organizations, etc.

If some members of your primary blood family are continually negative and not interested in helping themselves or others, then you may need to reconsider your relationship. You should continue to love them, but you don't need to be dragged down with them. You don't need to feel responsible for their happiness. No one should sacrifice their own peace and stability of mind by giving endlessly to a misguided and resentful blood family member simply because someone else or some blind tradition put that obligation on you. For some of us, these lessons are hard-learned, but better late than never.

The disgruntled family members may also be unhappy with the relationship they find themselves in with you. So, liberate them as you liberate yourself. Make their road to peace easier and also your own. Many people are probably held in unwelcome captivity by an ancient bondage that hinders their growth. This could go on forever if it weren't put to a test as serious as AD caregiving.

I can interact with my siblings now, and there is really no problem. There is no anger nor disagreements nor anything negative. What there is from my point of view is an absence of feeling—the positive, buoyant energy that we shared throughout our lives is gone. The amount of loss varies from one sibling to another. In other words, the depth of my feelings is different with each sister, depending on how far we've strayed from each other. I imagine each of them has a perspective on that same relationship with me. This is not a bad thing. This is honest, and as painful as that can be at times, still honesty is the best standard and allows you to know where you stand. Isn't that what everyone wants, simply to know where he or she stands?

I don't want to paint a negative view of my siblings. They are basically very nice people. They can be kind, essentially honest, generally gracious, and not prejudiced toward other people, regardless of the person's race, religion, physical or mental handicaps, etc. Those are very good qualities. We were raised with those standards. However, once a sibling establishes a separate "family" and allows himself or herself to be controlled by some person or dogma in that family, things can change shockingly with regard to his or her original family.

To their credit, most of my siblings have now made considerable personal recovery since their negative behavior during the issue of parental caregiving. I believe they're thinking more clearly now. I'm proud of them for that. I sincerely hope that progress continues.

*****

So, once a family member is forgiven, what does that bode for your future relationship? Do you return to family get-togethers and intertwine in each other's lives? Not necessarily. Again, the criteria for bonding after forgiveness depend on the health of the situation. If it aids your spiritual growth, then it can be positive. However, to return to the same situation without true change is just asking to be put through the grinder again. It is not advisable to maintain a family relationship that is unhealthy, for that would be masochistic. As the well-known saying goes, "Those who forget the lessons of the past are bound to relive them."

I've seen one of my sisters steadily throughout caregiving. Two others have wanted to get back together and just "put all of this behind us." The problem with just automatically putting it all behind us is what I described in the previous paragraph. So we move on.

If you find yourself in such a situation with your siblings, as perhaps millions of other caregivers have, accept that those things were bound to happen for whatever reason. If we can meet our siblings again on happier grounds—okay. If we can't—okay. We have to get on with our individual lives and be true to ourselves. As we grow beyond the negative portion of the crisis, the experience should be viewed as an opportunity for renewal and rebirth. Similar to the process of initial birth, a newborn leaves the comfort of the known for a whole new world. We may need to be forced into that change, but once there we become aware of the infinite possibilities awaiting us. Forgive your siblings, as you wish to be forgiven yourself. Remember the good times you've shared earlier in life and fix those in your mind. Then wish those people well and move on. It is really an act of love to liberate someone from an unhappy relationship.

I believe the will of God is to forgive. In my case, forgiveness is a big step on the road to understanding, happiness and serenity. And that's the road I'm traveling now.

CHAPTER 7

WORST NIGHTMARE— THE CATASTROPHIC EFFECT

If you learn from your suffering, and really come to understand the lesson you were taught, you might be able to
help someone else who's now in the phase you may have
just completed. Maybe that's what it's all about after all.
—Unknown

THE NEUROLOGIST LISTENED WITH RAPT ATTENTION AS I VIVIDLY
described the most sanity-threatening journey of my life—a four-
teen-hour drive with an Alzheimer's disease patient who was suffering a
psychotic breakdown. The doctor gave no indication that he wanted to
interrupt my account of the terror that Mother and I had been through.
Perhaps it was the manic tone of my voice as I was transported back to
the night while describing it all to him; or the unique circumstances
which allowed the episode to go on for so long and create such a rare
experience; whichever the reason, he wasn't about to move until he had
heard every word.

This office visit was taking place several days after our return to
Indianapolis—late April 1994. I had called Mother's primary care physician, and he had referred us to the neurologist. Now Mother was waiting
in another room as I gave a detailed description of a nightmare which is
beyond most people's comprehension.

After I finished speaking, the doctor said, "What you and your
mother experienced is called 'the Catastrophic Effect'." He went on to
say that the condition was not common, and the degree and duration of

our experience made it rare if not unique. It occurs when the world of the Alzheimer's patient falls completely apart. It is a full psychotic breakdown; at least it appeared to be that way in our case.

The neurologist gave me some emergency medication for her in the event anything similar should happen again though he didn't expect that we would need it. That is, we wouldn't be duplicating the circumstances which brought the episode on. However, there was the possibility that another situation could trigger it. As we were leaving his office, the doctor said to me with apparent sincerity, "If I can be of any help, please call me." How often do you hear that from a doctor? I believe he was truly moved.

I was still in shock from the recent experience on the long drive. Mother was unaware that the disaster had even taken place. Such is the fortunate side of AD—that brutal events can be quickly forgotten. Although in this case, the effects on her nervous system would take a couple of days to settle down. My recuperation would be much slower.

Before going further, I should start from the beginning to explain the horrible event. Also, I'll write of the conditions which set the stage for it all. Hopefully, our experience will help other caregivers and patients to avoid the circumstances and environment that are fertile grounds for producing such a disaster.

I have written this account from the notes I made at the time of the trip and shortly thereafter and portions I was able to write after some time had passed. Also, most of the elements of the journey—visions and emotions and endless details—are still with me, eleven years after it occurred.

Respite

Caregivers need a break—a respite. I believe that is true of all caregivers. However, in this case, I am speaking of primary caregivers for Alzheimer's patients. Personally, I'm speaking of my situation as primary caregiver for my mother.

In May 1992, I began to take a week a year to get away from home and go camping near the beach at a state park in Florida. It was okay to leave Mother alone at that point. She had friends and neighbors at the townhouse complex. Also, a good friend of mine would check on her. She also had my sisters' phone numbers if anything came up. I called her daily to make sure everything was okay. She told me things were fine, and I really didn't have to call each day, but I knew she was happy that I did. Her main symptoms then were "forgetfulness" and vulnerability to all the trials of any senior-age widow—a common one then being the endless calls of telemarketers aimed at the aged. She was still very functional. I made the same trip to Florida in May 1993. A week of camping and swimming in the Gulf of Mexico was great medicine.

In 1994, the AD had progressed to the point that I wasn't comfortable in leaving her alone. At the same time, that brief getaway was becoming increasingly important to my overall health and subsequent effectiveness as a caregiver. So, I asked my sisters to look after Mother during my absence. Their replies—"She wouldn't like it at our house," "There just isn't any room in our house," etc.—all added up to replies of "No." Nor would any of them come to Mother's townhouse to stay with her there. I didn't tell Mother any of this.

Finally, one or two of my siblings said that I should take her to Florida with me. My siblings had no knowledge of AD or chose not to acknowledge the diagnosis; nor did they have any idea of what caregiving entailed, nor of the need for caregiver respite. On top of that, they knew that I was going to be camping, certainly not a comfortable situation for Mother in her condition. Still, that was the only suggestion that was offered.

Another option was to put Mother in a nursing home for a week, as some caregivers did with their AD patient in order to get a respite. I didn't consider that an option at all. She would be quite conscious of having been put in a nursing home, and the effect on her morale would have been disastrous. Eventually she would have to go to a nursing home if she lived long enough, but I wouldn't do it just so I could have a rest.

Faced with the choice of taking Mother along or not going at all, I decided to ask her to come with me, and she agreed. I altered my attitude to see this in a positive light—we were good friends; we were both cheerful, optimistic people; and this would be her final chance to enjoy the Gulf beach which was reminiscent of our home long ago.

I had no idea of the disorientation and chaos that can happen to an Alzheimer's patient on a trip. I never read nor heard of the Catastrophic Effect or the more recent category termed catastrophic reactions. I had read a little about Sundowner's Syndrome, and we had experienced it some months previously. That happened when Mother and I were returning at dusk from a meal at my sister's who lived about twenty miles away. As darkness was slowly falling, Mother had made some comment about the light, and then said, "We have to get home." She made a few other related comments. I could hear and feel her increasing anxiety and knew that it had to be related to the AD. Her anxiety mounted until we were home and indoors. Fortunately it wasn't a long drive.

That was the Sundowner's experience that sticks most in my mind. What we were to experience with the Catastrophic Effect was at least a hundred times worse. By comparison, the Catastrophic Effect made Sundowner's Syndrome seem like a happy stroll in the Easter Parade.

Now, my principal concern was about getting some respite…some rest…getting away from caregiving and AD. That no longer was completely possible since I wouldn't be alone. Also, I would have to get a motel now, as camping would be out of the question. Still, I wanted to concentrate on the bright side of the trip. So, we packed and otherwise prepared. In the morning we were on the road.

*****

The drive started out well. We were in good spirits and ready for Florida. We were driving south on I-65, and it was a bright morning. At noon, after a couple of hours on the road, I noticed a puzzled look on Mother's face. I asked, "Anything wrong?" She looked disoriented, and asked, "Where are we going?" I explained about the trip and heading to Florida. She seemed to accept that, and we kept driving. Not long after that, she started asking again, "Where are we?" I explained, and we continued. Several hours into the trip, we were near Tennessee and her agitation was up again. I had to just keep talking to keep her at some ease. I decided to stop early that evening, or late afternoon. We were still in Tennessee, and I'd hoped to get further. I assumed her uneasiness was related to needing food to raise her blood sugar, and the fact that she hadn't taken a long drive for three or four years. After finding a motel, we went to have supper.

I made notes on different portions of the drive…usually within a couple hours after the incident. My records for that first day are as follows:

4/4/94, 6pm—Mother agitated, asks if we'll get back to Indianapolis tonight.

 7:15pm—Dinner. Before meal arrived, M was agitated about where we are, where we're going, [her] not having money, not having sufficient clothes. Tried to reassure her that we have enough of everything.

8:15pm—Back in motel room; NCAA championships on TV; she's very happy to see that. [TV basketball seems to reorient her back to home and safety.]

The rest of the night passed quietly and without incident, and I thought she'd be okay now. However, the following morning brought a new surprise. My notes for that are as follows:

4/5/94, up at 8am

 Mother asks, "Where is Heydon?"

I reply, "I'm Heydon."

"Well, yes, but the other Heydon."

"Dad?" My father had had the same name.

"Yes, I guess."

"He's dead. He passed away three years ago."

She didn't seem to hear or understand what I had said. She went on, "Okay, but where did the other man go?" and on…and on…

Now I had a lot to deal with. The confusion had not ended the night before as I had hoped. It seemed to be getting worse. Perhaps hardest of all was that this was the first time my mother was not able to recognize me. We had always been very close and now she didn't know—at least temporarily—who I was. Yet, there was so much to contend with that I couldn't dwell on that matter.

The following morning we continued south with no more general disorientation until noon or so. We were in northern Alabama when her questions cropped up again. I didn't know what I was in for. I wrote the following:

4/5/94, mid-day—M asked again where we are. Keeps trying to make sense out of nonsense. Frustrated w/inability to remember. Very tedious. Somewhat better after eating. It would be harder for someone else to handle this. Talk of the forest and Christmas trees. Often asking me, "Do you know where we are?"

We had crossed into Northern Florida from Alabama, and I figured we had a couple hours of travel left before reaching the beach. Her agitation was beginning again. I decided to stop for a bite to eat when we passed a small roadside park with a picnic table. We were on a back road, and it was quiet and peaceful. After eating we finished the drive and found a motel for the night at Panama City Beach. I continued:

Mother asks if we're going home tomorrow. I explain again about staying at the beach for a week once we find a spot we like.

4/6/94—Woke up at 7:30am. M wondered where we were. Abnormally cautious going down stairs as we were on the second floor. Stopped for coffee. Checked motels for vacancy. All motels full with college and high school students here for spring break. Drove west on 98A. Found nice motel on beach east of Pensacola to rent for a week—4/6/94-4/13/94.

4/7/94—M. is a little more comfortable. Sun is pleasant and relaxing. Dinner at Sam's restaurant. Crowded and noisy which upset [M.'s] balance a bit.

4/8/94 – Morning sun, good walk on the beach. [M.] a little unsteady on the sand. Drove to Milton. She spoke with old folks while I was at health food store/flea market. Beautiful day. [M.] was comfortable with the ride and back roads.

4/9/94, Noon—[M.] asked where the rest of the people are. "What people," I queried.

"The people who came with us," she replied. She won't elaborate on who those people are when I probe. (This is not the first time this subject has come up.)

4/9/94, 6pm – Went to dinner and then shopping.

"Where are we staying?" Mother asked.

"Here at the beach," I replied. "We're going back to Indiana on Wednesday."

"Are you coming to Indiana too?" she asked.

"Yes."

"Are you going to stay in Indiana?"

"Yes."

"Oh good," she smiled.

4/9/94, 9pm – "I think I better get back to Indiana," M. said.

"We're going on Wednesday," I answered.

"Are you going too?" she asked.

"Yes, we're both going."

"Oh. How are we getting there?" she asked.

"We're driving."

"Do you have a car?"

"Yes. It's the Tracer wagon—your car."

"Mine? Hmmm… I didn't bring any money."

"That's okay. I have enough for both of us," I said in trying to reassure her.

"Are you sure?" she asked.

"Yes."

And so on for another hour.

I noticed the next morning that her questions began to diminish. She was starting to feel more comfortable. Her security base had transferred to where we were staying. She still didn't realize where we were, but it didn't seem to matter so much as she mentally reestablished her sense of home to where we were staying. We enjoyed the sun and the gulf and some good seafood.

The night before we were to return to Indianapolis, I told Mother we'd be leaving the next morning, and that sounded fine to her. We did some packing that night and then had a pretty good sleep. (Mother always slept soundly, no matter where she was.)

Because she had adjusted to our new environment at the beach, I thought her discomfort was over and that the ride back to Indiana would be smooth sailing. If I had apprehensions about her stability during the return trip, they were beneath the surface. I was optimistic.

I had absolutely no idea of the hell storm of insanity that was coming our way. We were packed, somewhat rested, smiling and seemingly ready for the drive back. The utter chaos and terror of Alzheimer's roughest side was about to grow exponentially.

*****

Life is full of surprises, they say. Most of those surprises are not enough to shake up your world, to really get your attention. However, the big ones do.

When you're driving to work with a head full of preoccupations and plans for the future, and suddenly there is an earthquake, your mind is instantly cleared of what you believed was important. In a flash, every previous thought in your mind becomes irrelevant. It doesn't matter if you were planning your daughter's wedding or a loved one's burial or a joyous trip around the world; or, if you were facing an IRS audit or your house foreclosure or local evidence of African killer bees—suddenly it all drops by the wayside and you say, "What was that?! Am I in danger?! How can I survive this?!" There's nothing quite like an earthquake to get your undivided attention.

Another such shock would be that of a soldier who suddenly and unexpectedly comes under full attack. Every musing and other distraction quickly disappears and is replaced by panic or thoughts of how to respond and survive.

Those are the types of events that quickly threaten your physical safety, mental stability, and very existence. In that same vein, there are other actions that can seriously rattle your mental, emotional and spiritual stability prior to thoughts of physical survival. These include unknown conditions that you had never previously imagined nor even heard of.

*****

The first time your mother doesn't know who you are will definitely get your attention. When shock or dementia or the combination working together make you a stranger to her, your world can suddenly crumble. This is especially true if you have had a very positive relationship with her, if you normally laugh and joke together, as well as discuss the serious side of life.

For most people, mothers are the absolute cornerstone of any healthy nurturing in life, as well as representing any stability in this very unpredictable existence. Whether Capitalist or Communist, believer or atheist, a person will most often make their mother the anchor in this storm-tossed life. If anyone cares about us, it is our mother.

If the lack of recognition is the result of a progressive dementia, then you might be eased into that loss; that is, they forget you for a second but then rebound with a look or word that assures you that you're known again. Still, that loss of recognition is hard enough.

By studying the pattern of dementia in an AD patient, a person—especially a caregiver—learns to expect strange behavior. While caring for the AD patient, a caregiver makes note of the irregular pattern of the patient's decline. It is not a steady downward road. Most often it is two steps down and one back up. So, it is a downward development overall. On the other hand, parents raising children most often see the pattern of two steps up and one back, moving steadily forward and upward. Although the child-raising parent faces minor setbacks in training, he or she knows that the child is moving upward; further, that their nurturing is part of the process of helping the child to reach independence and maturity.

Caregivers for Alzheimer's patients may have minor victories, but ultimately they know that their loved one is sinking into advanced dementia and death.

*****

Now back to the subject at hand—the first time your mother doesn't recognize you. That had happened to me on the drive down to Florida. I don't remember that experience as being traumatic. I had so much to contend with at the time, including full responsibility for the welfare of this loved one who was experiencing some trauma from this serious neurological disease.

When you are on the first day of a lengthy trip (ten days, 2,000 driving miles) and your friend/navigator/other half doesn't recognize you, then it can be cause for some alarm. If that other person happens to be your mother—a gentle, helpful human whom you love and trust a great deal—then you could be in for some shock. Fortunately, that didn't throw me off much, at least as I remember it now. I'm a low-key and experienced person, and it usually takes quite a bit of chaos and threat to rattle me. Conversely, I can be worried by the seemingly easier task of adjusting to our ever-changing national economy.

On this return drive to Indiana, we were to face things far worse than Mother not recognizing me. A situation ten times worse than nonrecognition is when your mother not only doesn't recognize you but sees you as a potentially dangerous stranger.

Finally, I'll take you to a scenario which is ten times worse than the last. Not only does your mother see you as a threatening stranger, but the two of you are in a confined environment in the middle of nowhere in the middle of the night, and there is nowhere to escape nor possibility of help...for either of you. This last description is the experience I had. It was the most horrible and sanity-threatening experience of my life. It is extremely rare for an Alzheimer's caregiver to have to face this, since the circumstances were so singular. Mother's neurologist and a doctor at the VA encouraged me to write about it with the idea that it could be helpful to other AD caregivers, especially as a preventive measure; that is, that they may be aware of warning signs and also try to avoid a confined and alienated environment.

The young VA doctor was at the emergency room where I went just hours after the episode was over. VA doctors overall appeared then as a notoriously desensitized group—ask most veterans who went to the VA before 1995—and sometimes seemed to feel little accountability to their patients who were their captive audience. That's how my doctor was that day at the VA ER. He asked with apparent disinterest what was wrong. I told him the story and by the end his mouth had visibly dropped. It took a minute for him to collect himself. He wasn't detached any longer. He didn't stop me during the story, and the fact that I was still in manic mode just heightened all the details of the experience. Still, according to VA hierarchy, treatment was out of his realm so he had to refer me to another doctor to be seen the next day.

*****

I view the Catastrophic Effect as the psychotic condition resulting from an AD patient's world falling completely apart. It's probably one or two steps away from full madness, insanity, heart attack, or stroke. Essentially, the experience would be little different from that of an average person driving down the road and seeing in the distance the unmistakable form of a nuclear mushroom cloud, then thinking, "My God! That's it! Life's over!" Still, after the shock, and striving for survival above all, the person would seek some little bit of shelter, something to provide a sprig of hope. In the following case, the AD patient suffered extreme delusions for hour after hour, and a virtually constant sense of terror and impending doom. For me—the caregiver—it was a trauma of the most severe stress.

The day after this experience, I spoke with another doctor at the VA in order to decompress a little and hopefully get a sleeping tablet to help me get one night of rest. I was still wound pretty tight. After he had listened to my story, he said, "I've never heard of anything like that. I was on a trip once with a friend, and my brother was riding in the back-seat. My brother has some mental illness, and he was having an extreme manic episode. Still, that was nothing compared to what you went through." A partial account of what I did go through now follows.

The Drive

On the final morning of our Florida stay, I took a last swim and then packed the car. It was noon, and we were starting the ride back north to Indiana. I had some underlying anxiety about our return trip, though I had written off the earlier driving experience to low blood sugar or the shock of leaving our real home or some such reason.

Our route took us through a couple hours of the back roads of northern Florida and southern Alabama before linking up with I-65. The first hour was fine, but then the problem slowly began. Almost two hours into the trip, Mother started telling me, "We have to turn back." I asked, "Why?" She just repeated, "We have to turn back." After I asked her again, she said, "I forgot something." I assured her that I had checked every drawer, under the beds, on the porch, everywhere, and we had packed everything. To which she replied, "No, I forgot something." Then I asked, "What is it that you forgot?" She answered, "Just something. We have to turn back."

We were on I-65 at this point and over two hours into the drive. I explained again that I had packed everything, that there was no place to go back to since our time was up at the motel, and that we had to get home. I thought that she might be hungry and need a restroom, so I pulled off to a rest area about 3:30pm, and we had a little picnic of fresh fruits and sandwiches. The food and stretching the legs seemed to help a little bit, but she still appeared disoriented.

Back on the road, she started talking again about turning back. It was beginning to worry me, and the sun was going down. My hope was to get home as soon as possible and probably to drive straight through—the thought being that once she went to sleep I could just keep driving, and she would wake up when we got to Indianapolis. Her agitation increased until she was almost shouting, "We've got to turn around!" I knew I had to do something, as she couldn't be put off any-more. I finally agreed, "Okay, we're going to turn around and go back." Thinking that her increasing mania and disorientation might throw off her sense of direction, I decided to pull off at the next exit, take a left, drive a couple of blocks, turn around, and then get back on the onramp heading north again. When the next exit came into view, I told her, "We're getting off now." She quieted down but still was ill at ease. I tried my trick and got back on the north onramp; however, not long after I was on the road again, she started again, "We've got to turn around!" My patience was wearing down, and I said, "Mother, please stop this! We're going to have an accident." To which she screamed, "I'm not your mother!" Then I knew we had real trouble. She didn't know who I was, and she was scared. We would have to stop for the night. Hopefully some rest would mend her. The above statement, tell-ing her to stop or we would have an accident, was by far the strongest reaction I made to her during all the years of caregiving, before and after this trip. It showed that I was very tired, and for that one moment that I illogically believed she had some control over that behavior.

I pulled off at the next exit and followed a sign to a motel. It wasn't dark yet. I pulled up in front of the office, and said, "Okay. We'll stay here for the night." Her face turned to one of terror as she said, "No! I'm not that kind of girl!" Oh God help us, I thought. Now she not only didn't recognize me but further thought that I was a stranger who was a threat to her.

"What do you want to do?" I asked.

"We have to go back!" she replied.

"Okay," I said. Still, I decided to try the north onramp again in-stead of the southbound ramp she wanted. She didn't fall for it. Soon after, she started again with the building hysteria. "Just let me off! Let me off! Let me off!" she cried. I realized then that the only help for this was to go straight to a hospital emergency room. I said that we would be getting off at the next exit. Once off the highway, I pulled into a restau-rant/service station and asked the clerk where the nearest hospital was. There was one nearby he said and then gave me directions. I walked back out to the car resigned to a night in the hospital. Reaching the car, I opened the door, and Mother said, "Oh, there you are. Thank God!" My spirits were suddenly lifted. I thought that she had come to her senses and knew who I was.

Then she asked, "Did you see him in there?"

"Who?" I asked.

"The man who was driving me!" she cried.

It was time to think fast. "Yes, I believe I did see him. He's in the restroom in there."

"Oh no!" she cried.

"I won't let anyone hurt you," I replied.

"Let's go quickly!" she said. "Will you drive?"

"Sure," I said. I climbed back into my seat, started the car, and we turned into the onramp. I looked over and saw that she had bent her head down to the seat, so that she couldn't be seen. It was horrible to see her suffering this way.

She looked up at me and asked, "Do you see him?"

"No," I answered, "he's gone." Once we were on the road, I told her that it was okay to get up now, that she was safe and okay.

"Oh, thank you," she said.

"Who was that man?" I asked.

"I don't know," she said.

Anyway, I was so relieved and thought that we would be okay now. Some of the stress was leaving her face.

After a few miles, she asked, "Where are you driving?"

I told her that I was going to Indianapolis.

"Oh, me too!" she cried. "Would you give me a ride?" she continued.

"Yes, I'd be happy to," I replied.

"I don't have any money for gas," she said sadly.

"That's alright. I have plenty," I said. She seemed to relax and closed her eyes. Again, I thought that things would at least be calm now. By her comments, I could tell that she didn't know who I was but at least she saw me as a friendly presence.

*****

I stopped on the outskirts of Nashville to get some sandwiches and coffee. She awoke, and asked what we were doing. I explained. Now she seemed a little disoriented again. As we headed toward Louisville, she looked as though she was wondering again who I was. She just couldn't put any of it together. It was pitch black on this highway winding down through the mountains.

"Where are we going?" she asked.

"We're going to Indianapolis," I replied.

"You're going in the wrong direction," she said.

"No, this is right," I said. "We'll be in Louisville in a couple of hours."

The remaining drive to Louisville was filled with a building intensity of her fears, and it was very difficult. Much of the roadside was dark and undeveloped which probably aggravated her discomfort. My nerves were pretty frazzled, and I had to draw deep for inner strength to get me through this one. My thinking now was that once we got to Louisville she would make the connection with Indiana being just over the Ohio River. Further, that she would recall the short two-hour drive to Indianapolis.

We made it to Louisville at midnight. She quieted a little, perhaps feeling a little more secure with all the lights in the city and with the interstate cutting through it. Then we crossed the Ohio, saw the "Welcome to Indiana" sign, and I said, "See, we're back in Indiana now. We'll be home in two hours."

She didn't respond as I had hoped. She stayed quiet and the suspicious look was back on her face. About ten or fifteen miles out of Louisville and into Indiana countryside, the lights dropped away, and it was very dark. Her discomfort was growing again, as she said that Indiana was back the other way. The remaining two-hour drive was one of the absolute roughest times in my life. Every mile was truly like pulling teeth, as the old saying goes. It was pure torture. Her fear and hysteria were continuing to grow, and I didn't know if I could make it to Indianapolis. Still, there was no alternative, other than pulling to the side of the road and waiting for a highway patrolman and then an ambulance. Even that would probably have taken longer than getting back to Indianapolis. There was no way out. The only choice was to continue ahead.

She wanted me to stop the car. She wanted to turn around. She wanted to get out of the car. On and on the hysteria continued. I had to draw on my deepest reserves to get through it and keep the atmosphere from exploding. I had already driven for twelve hours when we got to Louisville, and ten of those hours had been under some of the most intense strain imaginable.

Finally, the lights of Indianapolis were visible, but they didn't register with her. I drove through the city and neighborhoods toward our home. She didn't recognize anything. She was still very upset, suspicious and scared. I knew then that we had to go to the hospital.

We pulled into the emergency room at Community North Hospital about 2:00 AM. Mother wouldn't get out of the car, fearing whatever. I went in and explained this to the triage nurse, and she reluctantly came outside with me. So we walked Mother inside, and they took her to an examining room while I waited. After an hour or so, they let me go in and see her. She smiled a little and said, "Where have you been?" I didn't know if she recognized me as her son now but at least she saw me as a friendly presence again.

The doctor gave Mother an injection of an anti-psychotic medication to help relax and restore her, but it didn't do much good in terms of really relaxing her. Normally, a dose of that medication would have knocked her out for days since she didn't take any medications and was of small physical stature. However, due to the state she was in when we arrived at the hospital, the medication barely slowed her down.

We got home about 7:00 AM. At the townhouse, we walked to the back porch and saw the sun coming up. She picked up her broom and started sweeping, finding order and peace in work as she always had. She was okay now—not restfully restored but grounded in her home and furnishings. She was not the least bit sleepy after having been awake for twenty-four hours and living through an incredible amount of stress in that time. The "blessing" of AD is that such an experience will quickly leave the patient's memory. She was in better shape than I was at that point. I was wrapped very tight. I tried to sleep but after a couple of hours of tossing and turning I gave up. My nerves felt raw the rest of the day. I was definitely tired but not sleepy. That's when I went to the VA as mentioned previously. Mother had a nap in the afternoon, as did I. We both turned in early that night.

She was much better the next morning, at least she was back to the stage of dementia where she had been before our trip. That is a "good" side of Alzheimer's—forgetting the bad things very quickly. As for me, the shock was slower to leave my consciousness. I was so thankful that it was over and that we made it through okay. However, the mark it left on me was a serious learning experience, and one that I wouldn't have to repeat.

A big consideration in our ability to survive that experience was that Mother and I were both very calm by nature, especially her. Also, we were both in very good physical health with strong hearts. If we had encountered that episode with anything less, I am sure we would not have made it through. Heart attack, stroke, nervous breakdown, something life-threatening would have claimed us. The reason the trip lasted so long—that I just didn't stop at a hospital later in the evening—is that she had given me enough hope on two or three occasions, when she saw me as a friendly presence, that I felt we could make it through okay. We almost didn't make it.

In the Alzheimer's Association literature, there is some reference now to an area called "catastrophic reactions." I read their info and didn't find anything like what we went through. Also, I've seen all the videos they have on the subject at the National Alzheimer's Association Library (Green-Field Library), and their reenactments don't begin to approach the severity of our experience. Our experience was probably singular due to the uncommon circumstances of our drive.

Other than this trip, the only other truly, consistently bad experience during my caregiving was the dissension in our family over the caregiving issue. That, also, is an experience I was reluctant to write about, but again, that would not be helpful to other current and potential caregivers who could, and probably will, be facing that most serious matter themselves.

In closing this accounting, I advise every Alzheimer's caregiver to carefully consider every trip you make with your patient. Whether it may be to the local bank or the doctor cross-town or to visit family across the state or country; whether it may be by car, bus or plane, weigh all considerations before making any trips away from the known, home environment. The advice of experienced caregivers and doctors may save you from life-threatening horror and the terrible anguish of the dreaded Catastrophic Effect.

CHAPTER 8

NURSING HOMES—
A MODERN, SAD REALITY

Over the hill to the poor-house—I can't quite make it clear!
Over the hill to the poor-house—it seems so horrid queer!
Many a step I've taken, a-toilin' to and fro,
But this is a sort of journey I never thought to go.

Strange how much we think of our blessed little ones!—
I'd have died for my daughters, I'd have died for my sons;
And God he made that rule of love, but when we're old and gray,
I've noticed it sometimes somehow fails to work the other way.

Over the hill to the poor-house—my child'rn dear, good-bye!
Many a night I've watched you when only God was nigh;
And God'll judge between us; but I will al'ays pray
That you shall never suffer the half that I do to-day!
—Will Carlton, 1867, *Over the Hill to the Poor-House*

NURSING HOMES ARE A SUBJECT THAT STRIKES DREAD OR TERROR IN the hearts of many millions of Americans, and with some justification. A feeling of total abandonment is the first perception, and then it just goes downhill from there. The older a person is, the stronger the apprehension of those facilities; one reason for that is the frightening history of the nursing home institution in America.

Before probing the subject of old age homes, I should mention that they are a much-needed institution in our current social structure. Without such facilities to take in the elderly disabled who have insufficient financial or human resources to care for themselves at home, our streets would be paved with elderly, disabled people. When I reached the point where it was impossible to take care of Mother any longer at home, she and I would have been in serious trouble without a facility to turn to. If a patient lives long enough, most every AD caregiver will face that painful action of having to release their care recipient to the care of someone else.

Considering Some Old Age Institutions

Before nursing homes, an older such institution in America was the "poor farm." The poor farm was for old people who had neither the family nor the financial means to survive on their own. At one point, it was also a dumping ground for orphans, widows, alcoholics, the mentally ill, and abandoned wives and children. When that institution took all the above groups, it may have gone by other names as well (e.g., the poor home, the county home, county farm, the almshouse).

Bernice would have learned about the poor farm from Grandma Pet or her mother, and that would have been the Whiteside, Illinois, poor farm at Round Grove Village, about 20 miles from Tampico. That's the poor farm that Ronald Reagan would also have heard about as a child since he lived in Tampico; I'm sure the reports affected him as they did my mother and anyone else who was warned about the possibility of ending up there. In those days of zero social safety net, prospects could change overnight with the loss of the family breadwinner, and people had to be aware of serious potential disaster.

I don't remember entering any nursing homes as a child. I don't believe there were any as we conceive of them now. There were "homes for the aged."

My initial vivid impression of a nursing home is from my first year of college at Indiana University (IU) extension in downtown Indianapolis. The period was the mid-1960s. The IU branch at that time consisted of three old buildings on the near-north side of the city. The buildings were interspersed with a few other old buildings—one being a nursing home. To call it a nursing home may be a stretch since it just appeared as rental rooms for the aged without any signs of medical personnel or equipment. The facility had a few rooms facing the street. Their windows were tall and nearly down to street level.

In attending a night class, I had to pass that building each Tuesday at 7:30 PM. Most times as I walked by, the curtains were open, and I'd see an old man or woman sitting or lying on a narrow, deeply sagging bed. The image that sticks with me is an old man with his head in his hands sitting on the side of the bed. The only light came from a weak, uncovered bulb hanging from an open wire that went into the ceiling. Old, faded wallpaper was peeling, and the low, yellow light made shadows on the dirty wall as the elderly man sat there in trousers and worn t-shirt. He looked truly despondent. I don't know if he could put thoughts together, but he appeared to be asking himself, "How did I get here? Is this what it means to be old? Did I really live?" I thought then as I do now that it was a very sad picture.

At this point some people might say, "Oh, no. That was long ago. Now we have more modern facilities and a lot of treatment regulations." Well, it's true that we have many newer buildings, though there are also still some older ones. It's also true that we have many regulations concerning resident treatment; however, that's not to say that all these regulations are followed and enforced.

What doesn't seem to have changed is the matter of heart and soul—how we feel and respond to our loved ones being in nursing homes; whether or not we visit, give them love, and try to bolster their spirits. Also, what hasn't changed is the fact that none of us want to end up in a nursing home. You can make as pretty a building as possible, but that will not make moving to such an institution more acceptable.

I've seen a lot of billboards and TV ads promoting various nursing homes. The portrayal of staff and residents always seems to be of happy, joyful residents and staff interacting as though they were at a party. After a total of nearly 3,000 visits to a dozen nursing homes, I have not commonly seen that spirit of joy in progress. If present, the joyful interaction is most likely to be displayed on holidays when residents' families are invited in for a party, or when an administrative person is showing a potential client around.

Life in nursing homes is not a problem for rich people. They can afford to have a round-the-clock staff of medical personnel come to their home to minister to their needs as they sleep in their own bed and watch the world go by. Nursing homes are not even a thought for them; that is, unless they fear their heirs may try to force them into one. How-

ever, that's another world; let's get back to the vast majority of us—
regular people facing this serious concern.

Mother, Dad, and Nursing Homes

Nursing homes are a mixed blessing. They provide some much-
needed relief for the caregiver, but they also represent an unknown in
terms of what care the loved one will receive. In choosing a nursing
home, I felt like a parent searching for the right day care center to guard
and protect my child. And, like a parent, I felt guilty that I had to leave
my loved one in the care of strangers.

Placing my mother in a nursing home was certainly one of the
hardest things I've had to do in this lifetime. Mother never showed fear
of anything as long as I'd known her and always overcame adversity with
a gentle strength, as well as faith and belief in the power of good. However, when the general mention of nursing homes came up eight or ten
years earlier, I saw her face drop, and she said solemnly, "I never want
to go there." She didn't elaborate on that, and I didn't ask.

What did these places represent to her? Born in 1913, she
wouldn't have seen any of them as she was growing up. She would have
seen, or known of, the county poor farm that was a symbol of elderly,
impoverished people who had no one to care for them. Actually, that's
the negative image; on a more positive note, she remembered that most
families took care of their elderly at home. That's what had happened
with her "Grandma Pet," her paternal grandmother who was perky and
optimistic and always made life fun.

Also, elderly family members staying at home would probably
have died at home, in the comfort of familiar surroundings and with
their loved ones present. That's another part of the cycle that has been
broken by modern life. My maternal grandmother lived with Mother and
Dad after her husband died, and then through her illness and death. So,
I believe Bernice felt that going to a nursing home meant that one was
being cast off, that a person placed in a nursing home was not really
loved by anyone or valued enough to be kept at home. And beyond the
abandonment, this just seemed to be something that was wrong, out of
the natural process.

My father had a horror of nursing homes as well—not so much
in fear as in a resolution that said, "I don't want to go there. I'd rather

die." Cut and dried. Earlier in this writing, I mentioned Dad's description of their neighbors going into a nursing home. It was almost as though he were describing innocent people being deported to a wasteland. That moment was the first time I had seen him seriously considering an infirm old age. Dad was then seventy-six, in failing health, and recognizing what was ahead of him. He was no longer the robust young warrior marching across Europe in a good cause and proving his metal. He was just another elderly human feeling his faculties diminish and wondering how his end would come.

The Nursing Home Decision

Putting your loved one—parent, spouse, or another person whose welfare has been entrusted to you—in a nursing home can be difficult beyond description. For me, it was simply heart-breaking. Six years ago—two and a half years after I had taken Mother to a nursing home—I wrote a column on choosing a nursing home. The column was published in the Indianapolis Star on April 5, 1998. Some statistics may be outdated, but there are some helpful tips in looking for a facility, so I've included the article below:

Shop around before choosing nursing homes for loved ones
By Heydon Buchanan (in "My Life" series)

Comes a time when the hard decisions have to be made. One of the hardest is if and when to place a loved one in a nursing home. That institution may go by other names like convalescent center or rehabilitation center, but they are all the same thing really.

When a person becomes a threat to themselves or others, a facility to help them must be considered. When the elderly and infirm face injury from a fall, or a fire from leaving the stove on, responsible action must be taken. I say "responsible," though the action is as much painful as responsible.

Not often is it socially considered a rehabilitation facility for the injured or ill, but in fact the vast majority of nursing home residents—perhaps to 75 percent—are taken to these facilities for rehabilitation.

This is not to say that the injured sent for rehabilitation are not also demented. Many people in some stage of Alzheimer's disease or other dementia have an injury that is the immediate problem that takes them there. Others need nursing care because of sickness resulting from malnutrition or dehydration.

Approximately 40 percent of the residents rehabilitate and then go home.

On the positive side, residents entering the nursing home nowadays for custodial care are much older than in earlier days.

People are living longer and living in their own home or with their family. Families are supporting their elderly longer. Meals-on-wheels and other services also help the elderly, housebound residents. Also, many people are in assisted living homes which are like a transitional step to the nursing home.

If I could give one piece of advice to families facing the nursing home dilemma, it would be to shop around beforehand.

Some folks are slow to think about nursing homes because they are in denial about their loved one's dementia, and where it leads.

Other people can't face the fact that they won't be able to care for their loved one at home; that, in fact, they must turn over that care to the nursing home—often fabled as the warehouse of death.

As a result of those reasons, as well as the unexpected illness and injuries which the elderly and infirm often face, approximately three out of ten families or guardians don't tour the nursing home before placing their loved one there.

Not touring the nursing facilities is very short sighted when you consider how much personal care your family member will need.

Nowadays, hospital stays are short. Commonly, social workers or "discharge planners" will call you from the hospital with the info that the doctor recommends a rehabilitation center and that you have two or three days to decide which one. After those two or three days, you will have to pay very expensive daily hospital rates, as your insurance will no longer cover any of the expense. That makes you move quickly.

The social worker may recommend some that are geographically desirable for you. However, quality-wise, it is your decision. And, to make an informed decision, you need to tour facilities.

To begin your search, you could ask friends and doctors if they have any recommendations. That will give you a starting point.

Also, before touring, make a list of your loved one's needs and your concerns. That info will make your interview time more efficient.

Here are a few items to consider on your arrival. Are you greeted politely by staff? Are the Director of Nursing and Chief Administrator personable and do they appear competent? (You will be having an extensive relationship with these people, so think about that during your visit.) Does the kitchen appear clean and sanitary? What activities are available for someone with your loved one's disabilities?

When you enter and tour the nursing home, keep your nose peeled for odors. There really should be none. There may be isolated cases, as that is part of the nature of incontinence, but it should certainly not be pervasive.

Another important feature is to check the nursing home's most recent inspection by the state. A copy of this report should be visible when you enter the nursing facility. Additionally, ask the Administrators about their last state inspection and what they have done to remedy their shortcomings.

After touring the facility with staff, you should make an additional tour of the nursing home during "off-hours" at your convenience. Evening time or on weekends, particularly during mealtimes—these are good periods to look the operation over at your leisure, without feeling rushed.

Nursing homes are nobody's idea of fun, but it's not the end of the world. Burning down the house is a lot worse. Also, being injured and not being able to call for help is a close second. Or, having an auto wreck and killing innocent people is a third.

Placing a loved one in a nursing home is a hard, hard call. However, in some cases of illness, injury and dementia, there is just no other choice.

One more piece of advice. If you do place a loved one in a nursing home, don't abandon them there. These people need love, probably more than at any time during their lives. The childhood lesson rings true, "Do unto others, as you would have them do unto you." (end of article)

While some statistics will have changed since I wrote that piece seven years ago, one part remains constant—putting your loved one in a nursing home never gets easier.

Being Forced into a Nursing Home Prematurely

In the block above, I wrote of nursing homes as an option when the caregiver is overwhelmed and can no longer effectively deliver care to their loved one. Everyone has a breaking point, and hopefully will recognize it before they end up in a hospital themselves. At that point, they can't serve their loved one or themselves.

There is another approach to the caregiving dilemma whereby the elderly parent, or ward, is put into a nursing home prematurely—premature in the respect that the family's motive for placement is more selfish. Such placement may be motivated by various reasons; however, two principal ones that come to mind are convenience and financial gain.

These two motivations are certainly not new, especially the matter of financial gain. The financial consideration could be related to the saying "Money is the root of all evil." That has been portrayed in some films showing the effort to put an eccentric old uncle in an institution in order to take over his estate.

Recently I read a poem from the nineteenth century that encapsulated both motives of this situation, as well as some additional selfish reasons for abandoning a parent to an institution. The poem is "Over the Hill to the Poor-House," written by Will Carlton in 1867. This poem and others by Mr. Carlton were inspired by the residents of the poorhouse at Hillsdale, Michigan. That poorhouse was in operation from 1854 until 1867 when it burned down.

Over the Hill to the Poor-House tells the story of a seventy-year-old widow who is healthy and ready to work for her keep but instead finds herself abandoned by her children and their subsequent families. She and her husband worked hard to raise their six kids and make sure they had what they needed to live and also go to school. That included a lot of love, joy, and sacrifice. Now her husband is dead, and five of the six kids have families of their own. She devotes herself to her final son at home. Then he gets married and brings his wife home. The wife is a snob and considers the mother uneducated, and ultimately leads the son to send his mother packing. The mother is terribly hurt, and then each of her other grown children comes up with excuses to not have her living in their homes as well. The mother says, "I'd have died for my daughters, and I'd have died for my sons. And God He made that rule of love; but when we're old and gray I've noticed it sometimes, somehow, fails to work the other way."

The Mother was shocked and confused by all the rejection, but she kept going in life. She then said, "So they have shirked and slighted me, an' shifted me about—so they have well nigh soured me, an' wore my old heart out; but still I've borne up pretty well, an' wasn't much put down, till Charley went to the poor-master, an' put me on the town! Over the hill to the poor-house—my child'rn dear, good-bye! Many a night I've watched you when only God was nigh; and God'll judge between us; but I will al'ays pray that you shall never suffer the half that I do to-day!"

This poem gained a lot of national attention. There was some negative response to the poem, and that may have been by people who didn't want to face the situation; or it may have been by people who had disposed of a parent in that way. In any event, the poem played a part in the passing of the Social Security legislation in the 1930s.

The combination of this poem plus awareness of everyone's local poorhouse or poor farm, and knowledge of neighbors or fellow residents who ended up in one of those institutions, put a fear in people about what their future might hold. I'm sure that Mother was very aware of these possibilities for everyone; and, as her mind fell victim to AD, I'm sure those images of old people being abandoned began to take on more weight.

I remember especially in some older Hollywood films when the dialog included the dramatic line: "What are you trying to do?! Put me in the poorhouse?!" The line usually came from a husband who felt his wife was overspending.

It's not my place to judge anyone for their decision in placing a parent/relation/ward/loved one in a nursing care facility; at rope's end, I had to do it myself. Every case is individual and with its own circumstances. That being said, I would suggest that people consider several factors before such placement: 1) Know that this is a major decision and will probably exist in your psyche until the day you die; 2) Reflect on "Do unto others as you would have them do unto you"; and 3) Know that your decision and motives will be seen and weighed by your children, other family members, and friends.

As I write this line, former President Reagan is less than twenty-four hours away from his funeral service in Washington, D.C. He is the nation's most famous Alzheimer's patient/victim. How coincidental that he and Mother's family came from the same tiny Midwestern town; he and Mother were born and died within two years of each other; and both were victims of Alzheimer's disease. However, the issue of nursing homes is not relevant to Mr. Reagan since there was medical support and other outside resources to allow him to stay at his home. I'm sure Mrs. Reagan would join me in showing admiration and great respect for the legions of AD primary caregivers who don't have such support and often sweat blood in order to take care of their loved ones at home as long as possible.

*****

As I write now, Mr. Reagan has been buried. My sympathies go out to Nancy Reagan as another person who has lost a much-loved person to Alzheimer's disease. Perhaps it's good that Mr. Reagan's case of Alzheimer's was made public if it draws more attention to the disease. It is a reminder that our society is so often celebrity-oriented. A week after Mr. Reagan was buried, I happened to make a new acquaintance, and we spoke about our lives and what we had been doing recently. When I told him about my personal experience with caregiving, he said, "So you've experienced some of what Nancy Reagan went through."

"Yes," I replied, "we've both lost a loved one to Alzheimer's disease. However, for the sake of accuracy, I would say that Nancy Reagan experienced some of what I went through."

Entering a Nursing Home

Concerning the technical part of entering a nursing home, I'll note some general information here since each facility will probably have additional criteria for being accepted as a resident.

There are two locations from which to enter a nursing home—from a private home or a hospital.

A potential resident can voluntarily enter a facility or be sent there by their guardian or Health Care Representative. Volunteer entrants are most commonly individuals with chronic health conditions who do not have someone to take care of them at home.

There is a screening by the nursing home to determine if they "can meet the resident's needs." The equal but undeclared purpose of this screening is to see if the potential resident meets the facility's needs and desires as well For example, how will the resident pay for the facility services? Can they pay in funds without using Medicaid? Is the patient mentally and emotionally stable enough—with medications if needed—not to be dangerous to anyone including himself or herself? This last query is especially appropriate in Indiana since the state mental hospital for central Indiana was closed, and some mental patients have been absorbed into the nursing home population.

There is also a pre-screening interview by someone representing the Council on Aging. This is to insure that an elderly person is not just being dumped into the nursing home system.

Nursing Home Deaths and Memorials

Any person who enters a nursing home as a long-term resident is going to die either there, or in a hospital if a health emergency arises. That's a serious thought for the new initiate—hopefully, dementia has set in by that point, and the place of death is not another grim consideration to be handled after the shock of coming to their new home.

I saw a number of deaths at nursing homes. Sometimes I didn't learn about a death until weeks afterwards when I'd ask about a resident I hadn't seen for awhile. Then I'd be told that he or she had passed away. In order to respect the family's privacy, deaths were not announced or posted in any way. Also, some nursing homes don't like to publicize any reference to death, as they consider it demoralizing.

Sometimes I'd be more aware of a death if the resident had been sick and confined to his or her room—that is, as opposed to a sudden dying and disappearance. At that point, I asked the nurse if it was okay to visit the person, or if the family had requested privacy. I went to a number of funeral callings, generally to express condolences to the surviving family members whom I'd known through visits in the facility or as other members of the Family Council—an organization I'll cover in more detail in the following chapter.

I watched two of my mother's roommates die. The second was a lady I'd known for three years. Helen was a sweet, little, old lady who could be feisty at times, but only when she was agitated due to confusion. She was ninety-six years old, weighed about eighty-five pounds, and her mind was generally clear.

Although I had gone in to see my mother, who was in bed and nursing a respiratory infection, I noticed around the curtain the darkness and a young cleaning staff employee named Marissa who had tears running down her face while she held Helen's hand. It was especially poignant to me since Marissa didn't speak English, and her compassion was truly based on one person to another at perhaps the most important point in life. We spoke in Spanish, and I was then told that Helen was close to death. She had an oxygen tube in her nose and was conscious and coherent and not really fearful, other than asking the young lady not to leave. I stayed with them and spoke to Helen about how I'd enjoyed our friendship over the last three years. She was smiling and holding my hand, and Marissa's hand in her other hand. After an hour or so, I stood up, kissed her forehead, told her I loved her, and that I would see her later.

The next morning I returned, and she was still alive. Helen's daughter and a close friend were with her, sharing smiles and love and talk of the life awaiting her, according to her faith. A priest had been in earlier to give last rites. Every so often, Helen would turn her head and look beyond her daughter, opening her arms and smiling as she did so. It was as though she was waiting to be lifted up and could see someone coming for her. I wasn't close enough to tell if she spoke some name.

Standing nearby, I gave Helen words of greeting. She stared at me but couldn't make a connection. I believe her recognition came and went, since the day before she thought Marissa was her daughter at one point. I pressed closer to her and suddenly a big grin went across her face. "Hi, sweetie," she said. Again I took her hand, kissed her forehead, and told her I loved her.

Marissa came by again that morning, so Helen had four of us standing by her bed and doing whatever we could to offer her comfort. She was smiling, and the scene was close to what many of us would want at the end of our lives, at least in terms of the human support and good feelings that attended. For choice of locale, I would idealize some beautiful setting in nature but that is incidental. Most important is the atmosphere. I believe that is controlled by personal acceptance of one's destiny. Helen's acceptance and anticipation of life to come were supplemented by the love surrounding her in that room.

Helen passed away later in the day. She was at peace and ready to bid farewell to this world.

*****

It wouldn't serve to describe all of the visitations and funerals I've attended related to the passing of friends at the nursing home. However, I believe one case in particular should be mentioned to make a point.

This service was a memorial being held at the nursing home prior to burial. There were at least a hundred people in attendance—family and friends, and perhaps other connections considering that this lady was involved in local politics. Ester had lived over ninety years and seen a great deal of change in the city of Indianapolis.

I knew Ester for about four years of her stay at the facility. While visiting Mother, I would stop by Ester's wheelchair and say hello and pat her shoulder. Or I would say, "I saw Tom (her son) today, and he said he'll be here later." And she would smile slightly, with her eyelids barely open, and say, "Oh thank you, thank you."

Anyway, at Ester's memorial, her minister said a few words to start the service and then restated that this was a memorial service so the family and friends in attendance were invited to come to the podium and express their memories of Ester as well. Her son stood up and went to the podium. He spoke very touchingly of being glad that he had overcome a personal problem for the last couple of years and how he had been able to help Ester as a secondary caregiver during that time. He went on to explain the contact and connection they had made during that period.

I thought he should be recognized for his faithful attendance to visit his mother at the nursing home. So, I planned to go to the podium myself to compliment him and also to speak of my interaction with his mother. I would wait until her family and friends had spoken and then walk up.

He finished his short comments and went to sit down. I waited for the next person to get up. Nothing happened for a minute, and I assumed that everyone was a bit reticent. Another moment passed, and then I thought I might as well be next. As I started to rise from my seat in the back, the minister came back to the podium and said, "Well, I know that Ester would be very happy to know that all of you have come to be with her today." He seemed a little confused or taken aback that no one else had gotten up to speak.

It was over. I couldn't believe it. Truly the minister had waited a sufficient amount of time, to the point where it was becoming a little awkward. However, I just couldn't believe that no one else had stood up to speak. Here, I, as a relative stranger, was going to talk but no one else did. Offspring, siblings, grandchildren, and other friends were all in attendance; yet no one spoke.

Afterward, I considered this and thought maybe the silence wasn't really so strange. I hadn't seen any of these people at the nursing home, other than her son. Perhaps some had visited her at the home, but I don't think so. I had seen a couple of people there once for a birthday party, but that was it.

Two ideas came to mind about this incident. First was the thought of how seldom many residents ever have a visit by family or friends. Secondly, I was curious as to why so many people would come to a person's funeral and yet not visit them in the nursing home, nor stand at a memorial and speak of the good qualities of the deceased or a meaningful experience they had shared with this departed loved one. On reflection, I do remember the group in attendance as being very staid, showing no emotion—no joy in remembrance nor sorrow at the passing of this presumed loved one they had come to bury. So, I came to believe that this memorial and burial were simply ceremonial formalities. It was probably protocol to be there. Perhaps Ester would have been the same at any of their funerals. Still, it was strange.

After the passing of my mother, I reflected on the difference of the two memorials. We had a much smaller number of people in attendance—Mother had outlived most of her friends—but we had more people speaking about her and her very special qualities.

I thought again about how visiting loved ones at the nursing home is critically important, far more important than whether they attend the person's funeral or not. And the important factor is not just making an occasional appearance; it is showing some real care. The people who have loved you are desperately in need of love themselves then. They need hugs and kisses and being told that they are loved.

*****

A couple of years ago, I was at a somewhat upscale wedding reception. Two middle-aged women, who apparently were friends and hadn't seen each for years, were standing behind me and catching up on their lives. The first lady completed her family review. Then the second lady talked about how her husband's career was going; how her son was in this school or that; a daughter was engaged and plans being made for the wedding; a younger son was playing football now; and she and her husband were making early retirement plans to travel here and there as soon as retirement came. She finished speaking, and then after a minute's pause she added as a brief afterthought, "Oh and we're also doing the nursing home thing."

I thought to myself, "The nursing home thing? What is that?" She had said it as though it was a common term, like saying, "We go out for coffee." Her mention sounded very vague and impersonal—the most minor of afterthoughts that she just happened to remember. Did it just mean they know someone in a nursing home, and they called once in a while to see how that person was doing? Or, did it mean that one of her, or her husband's, parents was in a facility and they occasionally stopped by to see him or her? To someone who was very involved in his loved one's care and was also a daily visitor, the term sounded very strange. For the sake of America's soul, I hope that term—the nursing home thing—does not become part of the nation's vocabulary.

*****

Nursing homes across the country are in a bad way in terms of providing a stable, good quality of life to their residents. Ninety percent of the nation's nursing homes are understaffed according to a recent federal study.[1] They also have extremely high staff turnover rates which result in ever-new personnel not knowing the patients; and the nursing home image is that of a dismal environment. The term nursing home is near universal in giving an impression of a hopeless and depressing situation.

The above article citing the federal study continues, "But the Bush administration, citing the costs involved, says it has no plans to set minimum staffing levels for nursing homes, hoping instead that the problem will be resolved through market forces and more efficient use of existing nurses and nurse's aides...."[2]

More efficient use of existing nurses and nurses' aides. I know many nurses and nurses' aides who would consider the President's comment to be a cold and callous insult, not to mention being simply stupid and uninformed. I'll provide details here. The many nurses I've known at nursing homes are already overworked and the nurse's assistants even more so. The doctor who was a co-author of the federal report said the recommendations would be for one aide or nursing assistant to have five or six residents from 7 AM to 11 PM. The current average in nursing homes during that time frame is one aide for every eight to fourteen residents.[3] The Certified Nursing Assistants (CNAs) are already responsible for roughly twice the number of patients as recommended by the federal report. If the CNAs get any more "efficient," the patients may have to change themselves.

How will the "market forces" improve the staff-to-patient ratio? Does the family member say, "Oh, my loved one isn't getting proper care? We'll leave here and go shop for another nursing home." I don't think so since nine out of ten nursing homes are understaffed. Even then, many don't have beds available; it's a captive market. Also, choosing a nursing home is a big process; and, changing nursing homes is a big process. And what of the multitude of disabled residents who have been abandoned to nursing homes and no one either visits or cares about them? What will the market forces do for them?

So, one out of ten nursing homes is adequately staffed according to the report. The last figures I saw on the socioeconomic breakdown of Americans showed that about nine or ten percent, or one out of ten people, is in the upper middle class. So, it's not too big a stretch to figure that the adequately staffed nursing homes (i.e., one out of ten nursing homes) are for the upper middle class citizens, one out of ten Americans. Those would probably be the nursing homes that also require cash payment and don't accept Medicaid designation.

What about the rich—the wealthiest one percent of Americans? Well, they probably will never see a nursing home. They will stay at their estate, or wherever they want to be, with a private medical staff to cater to their needs. They will have a one-to-one staff-to-patient ratio. You can't beat that.

President Bush could have been more candid and direct in his answer by saying to the reporter, "Look, I'm rich, and the matter of staff-to-patient ratio in nursing homes doesn't affect me, nor does it interest me at all. I'll be at home, coddled and pampered for the remainder of my life. Beyond that, I'll have the Secret Service as my bodyguards until the day I die. I have absolutely no interest in nursing homes or the frailties and vulnerabilities of old age as experienced by the vast majority of Americans." But I just don't think he'll be that candid. This may sound a little harsh to the uninitiated, but to a caregiver who has accumulated substantial experience working with nursing homes, our president's attitude sounds cold and indifferent. As mentioned previously, I've made thousands of trips to nursing homes, and I can't help but wonder how many times President Bush has visited them; or even been to one, other than to possibly shop for some votes.

Speaking of visiting a loved one at a nursing home, it's often nice to go in the evening after he or she has been put to bed but before the patient has gone to sleep. AD patients are often more relaxed then since the daytime stimuli of people, movement, and sounds have calmed down; thus, the AD patient is more at ease. I should add that some AD patients whose clocks are reversed are more awake at night instead of during the day. It all depends on the sleep pattern of your loved one.

*****

In America we simply don't want to think of old age, decay and death. It is just not a part of our life cycle thoughts. When people get old, they just disappear, not only in body but in stature and any relevance, except to be hauled out for family gatherings once or twice a year. At that point families can demonstrate that they do care about the aged members of their clan, at least as long as it takes to shoot a few family photos and finish that Thanksgiving meal. Then it's time for the old folks to go back into hiding. Maybe I'm being a little harsh but compared to the many civilized societies who respect and honor the elderly, our society gets a bad report card.

Having watched a number of folks transitioning into old age, I have heard the refrain from many seniors, "People should respect us." However, those same people may have avoided consideration of the elderly when they were younger, so nothing was ever done to alter society's thinking.

CHAPTER 9

NURSING HOMES—
ONE, TWO, THREE

Old age is the most unexpected of all the things that
happen to a man.
   —Leon Trotsky

Few people know how to be old.
   —François de la Rochefoucauld

In youth we run into difficulties; in old age difficulties
run into us.
   —Josh Billings

Old age ain't no place for sissies.
   —Henry Louis Mencken

BEYOND THE STRUCTURE OF THE NURSING HOME ORGANIZATION,
and the administrative requirements for becoming a resident, there
is the personal side—the day-to-day life that residents and their families
must work with. Residents have to live it on-site while family members
need to monitor it during their visits, to make sure the patient care
measures up to the services agreed upon.

During the span of seven-plus years, Mother was in three differ-
ent nursing homes—the first two on a temporary basis, as it turned out.
In covering those years, I will simply refer to the facilities as NH #1,
NH #2, and NH #3.

NH #1

There are two ways to become a nursing home resident—by choice of the resident or guardian, or through medical necessity as ordered by the patient's doctor.

Mother would never choose to enter a nursing home, and I would never take her to one as long as I was able to take care of her at home. If she had a serious injury or advanced illness set in, we might not have a choice in the matter. Also, if a patient lives long enough, and you are a primary and solitary caregiver, you will need the help of a nursing home at some point. My prayer was that none of those conditions might occur until her mind could no longer understand what was going on, so that she wouldn't experience that heartbreak of feeling abandoned in the nursing home.

Another of the issues that make Alzheimer's disease caregiving so difficult is the way the patient's cognitive abilities can bounce back and forth—one minute the patient appears to have declined to the point of not knowing what's going on, and then soon after, the patient is well aware of things. That adds another layer to the emotional pain of patient placement in a facility if the caregiver is concerned about the patient realizing what is taking place.

*****

On October 31, 1994, Mother had a transient ischemic attack (TIA) or mini-stroke. I called for the ambulance, and they took her to the hospital. On her second day there, she was stable, and her doctor ordered a stay in the convalescent/rehabilitation center, which translates to nursing home.

I learned of the doctor's decision from the discharge planner at the hospital. He called with the information, and then told me that I would have three days to find a nursing home for Mother. After November 4, she would be charged the full hospital day rate—some incredible amount of money. I had to find a place very quickly.

There was so much to contend with at once—realization, acceptance, and action. First was her medical condition itself—TIA plus Alzheimer's. Second, there was the idea—now reality—that Mother had to go to a nursing home, at least temporarily. Third, the nursing home had to be chosen and paperwork done within three days. And finally, that I was alone in having to get all this done. It was a heavy load.

As Mother's Health Care Representative, it was all up to me. I had no experience in this area. I had visited people in two different homes long ago, but I was in and out without looking around very much. How does a person choose a nursing home? I later wrote about that in my earlier published article as reprinted in the previous chapter. So, when you do decide on a nursing home, what if there are no beds available when you need one?

My oldest sister did join me in touring one of them, and in the end that was the one I chose. It was centrally located where family members could visit more easily during her stay. I didn't know how long that stay would be, for it was dependent on the doctor's release orders. There had been two other facilities which appeared better than the chosen one, but neither of them had any empty beds.

From the beginning, Mother was asking me to take her home. At this point, she understood when I told her that we had to wait for the doctor's permission. At least she understood it when I was talking to her. A few minutes later she would ask me again about going home. Mother had a strong body, and it was repairing itself. Also, I took her walking during my daily visits. In addition, she had some therapy when I wasn't there.

The facility itself turned out to be not very good. Too often the smells of urine were evident, and the patients were unkempt. The dining room was loud with some rowdy patients who should have been medicated or at least segregated. Loud outbursts are disturbing to anyone, particularly at mealtime; however, to the fragile elderly who are extra sensitive, the sounds are intensified and much more upsetting.

I can picture her room and first roommate there. There wasn't even a partition between the beds; perhaps there was a light curtain that just wasn't pulled. The roommate was a very old woman—apparently near death with her eyes closed and breathing through her mouth which was formed in an "O" shape with lips pressed out as though she was trying to whistle. I saw her a couple of times when I was visiting Mother, and then the declining roommate disappeared.

Now it was mid-December. Mother was better but still fragile. Her doctor was concerned that at home she wouldn't have the support of attendants around all the time to help her stand and generally take care of herself. I couldn't be around twenty-four hours a day, and my taking her to the bathroom was something neither one of us was ready for. If asked, Mother would have said, "No, I'm fine. I can go to the bathroom by myself." Or "I can walk upstairs by myself." The big change here was that Mother wasn't able to judge the level of her disability. At this point, her medical fate would be determined by her doctor and me—her Health Care Representative. Still, I would do my best to get her what I knew she wanted.

There was absolutely no home health care available through her medical insurance or Medicare. For some unexplained reason, the insurance companies and the government would rather pay for someone's stay in the nursing home than to provide a home health aide for a few hours a day. It would be cheaper for the insurance company and much more comfortable for the patient to be in his or her own home; however, it was simply not allowed. So, any supplementary help at home would have to be paid for by the family—net dollars, cash. At that time, home health aides cost $12 or $13 an hour through an agency, and that seemed prohibitive. Since there was no family support, I was totally on my own. It was simply Mother and me against the world. And it was a very big world with a long list of obstacles.

I began to imagine how a single mother without a supporting family must have felt during the Depression. During that period there was no Social Security, no Medicare, no Medicaid, no ADC (Aid to Dependent Children), and no family shelters. There were also no jobs and even if by the most remote chance the mother might get a job, there would be no one to watch the children, the babies, while she was at work. Many children were placed in orphanages as the only solution. Many were placed in the fraternal society version of an orphanage (e.g., the Masonic Home). What Mother and I faced was not so different; in our case, the option was a nursing home instead of an orphanage.

The family resistance alone was enough to tear my soul apart. Most of my siblings were suddenly at odds with me. They wanted Mother to stay permanently in a nursing home. I wanted her to have what she wanted and be able to come home. I was willing to do the work necessary to make that happen. I didn't tell her what they wanted, nor to my knowledge did they tell her. I doubt if they could tell her, for they must have known it would break her heart. Still, that was a severe emotional bout for me at the same time that I had to concentrate on Mother's care.

*****

By now, it was approaching Christmas. Mother was much better overall but still needed support with her walking. She was still asking me every day to take her home. She would ask softly and hopefully. When I mentioned the need for the doctor's okay, she would stop for a while. However, I knew that inside she was suffering emotionally.

One day I had a care plan meeting with the staff. A representative from each of the patient care branches attended to discuss Mother's treatment at the facility with me. That's where I met the Director of Nursing (DON) mentioned earlier who was also a primary and solitary caregiver.

The therapy area of a nursing home can be very profitable. During November 1994, Mother had some therapy on fourteen days of the month. The bill was over $10,000. As I remember, physical therapy cost $128.00 an hour, and speech and occupational therapy were about $164.00 an hour. Mother's savings could be used very quickly at that rate of depletion. She was still anxious to come home, so I arranged a home assessment by the therapists to tell me what needed to be done.

On Monday, December 19, 1994, I brought Mother to the townhouse for a home visit. The occupational and speech therapists joined us at home to evaluate the environment. Their recorded chart notes of that visit: "12/19/94—Patient (Pt.) seemed comfortable at home, more relaxed & less confused. Able to verbalize & point out living areas (e.g., kitchen, dining room, living room, bedroom, bathroom, television). Pt. demonstrated stability on carpeted services but needs some support at all times for safety. Able to do sit and stand with proper hand placements & sequencing, being stable almost 100% of the time. Toilet transfers are with some support for safety but she was able to perform proper maneuvers. Able to go up and down stairs…no difficulty assessed with activity & seemed to be in full control for sequencing. Talked with Heydon (son) about recommendations for more safe mobility around home.... Pt. then spent more time at home with son."

The following day, 12/20/94, the speech therapist noted in Mother's medical chart her first words to him: "I want to go home now."

For my part, I worked on getting assistive devices installed and shopping for home health aides. The aides would definitely be needed now since it would be impossible for me to do it all alone. The doctor had ordered 24-hour care, so I would have the aides work twelve hours a day in caring for Mother at home, and I would work the other twelve hours which included the night. Outside aides would be expensive, but less than the cost of a nursing home; and Mother would be able to stay home and sleep in her own bed. Bernice had some money to carry the expense for awhile. It was her money; and she wanted more than any-thing to go home. So, I decided to grant her wish and bring her home. Finally, I spoke with Mother's doctor, got him a copy of the therapists' report, and told him of the arrangement with supplementary aides. He agreed to her release.

Then I informed my sisters of my decision as her Health Care Representative. Some disagreed with the choice. Some may have had other plans for her assets. Although my sisters were not involved in her care—other than the Power of Attorney (POA) who wrote Mother's monthly checks—I had listened to their opinions before making my decision.

*****

In January 1995, after nearly two months in NH #1, I brought Mother home. In addition to the aides, I had the maintenance man at the townhouse put up all the support bars that the physical therapist at NH #1 had suggested. Everything was in place. For Christmas 1994, I had gotten a "pass" to bring Mother home from the nursing home for a day, but now we were checking out of NH #1 for good. It was a happy time for us as we climbed into the truck and laughed our way home.

*****

Bernice was so joyous upon arriving home. Her physical abilities were back to normal though her mental faculties were still slipping away bit by bit. In private, she kept telling me that she didn't need the aides around. She could do everything for herself, and that there was no need for that expense. I told her the doctor wanted it for a while anyway. My hope was that she'd just get used to them because the doctor wasn't go-ing to change the orders. Her condition was degenerative and progres-sive, but she couldn't have understood that.

As time passed, and her confusion mounted, she began to forget why the aides were there. That was followed by not believing she was in her own home. If I was upstairs or out doing errands, she would usually ask where I was. When I was out of sight, she was less grounded.

Her anxiety, anguish, and wanting "to go home" came more into play at this point. For the last eight months of her life at home, these pains and severe stresses occurred to some extent daily. I learned this again as I reviewed my notes from the period, as well as the daily notes made by the home aides I had hired.

As a most poignant example of the confusion Bernice suffered during that period, I will reference a journal note from one of the aides: "*Apr. 6, '95, 7:00 am, Bernice already up & in bathroom. Was shocked to see me & told me to leave while she gets dressed. Got very upset when I attempted to talk to her. Still insisting that I go – she woke Heydon to have him tell me. When he explained who I am she returned to her room & sat and cried. Refusing to get dressed just sitting.*"

I chose the above example because it encapsulates so much of the AD patient's frustration during this period of the disease. However, the condition was worse in the nursing home where she was even more exposed to strangers handling her, especially with the extremely high turnover rate of CNAs (Certified Nursing Assistants).

Concerning the above episode, imagine what it was like for this gentle lady who faced the disintegration of her mind and all these other changes happening to her as well. Try to put yourself in the mind of an AD patient. A stranger walks in on you in the bathroom in your home; not only that, but they just stand there and talk to you...ask you if you're ready for a bath. Then you call for the only anchor you have in life—the only person you can really trust—and he says that the doctor wants this stranger here to help you. Your sense of self and independent world have truly crumbled. All those experiences at the same time must have been horribly painful.

Bernice didn't understand or accept that we needed an aide to be with her for her own safety. She couldn't comprehend that the doctor had ordered it; nor would she have accepted the doctor's order with regard to life in her own home. Though she respected the medical profession and her doctor's "orders," infringing on her freedom at home was another matter. I explained things to her one minute, and the next minute it was literally gone.

We could have left the nursing home A.M.A. (Against Medical Advice) at any point, but that wouldn't have been helpful in any way. The outside aides were absolutely necessary to successful home caregiving for at least some period, and I agreed with the doctor. Also, to leave the nursing home A.M.A. would have gone against me at a guardianship hearing which still lay ahead of us then. Mother couldn't understand those matters even if I had tried to explain the A.M.A. and guardianship issues. She just wanted to be at home without outsiders trying to control and infringe upon her life.

So, in her frustration, Bernice went into her room and sat and cried. She must have been thinking in some way—"How did all this happen to me?"

I saw her reaction, and it pained me terribly. If anyone deserved a break at the end of her life, it was my mother. She did everything right, and that was a strange payoff. So, there was no question that any Divine plan was simply beyond human comprehension—at least beyond Mother's and my comprehension.

It was a horrible dilemma for me. Mother was terrified of nursing homes, and I had promised to take care of her at home. However, her increasing anguish was so painful for both of us that I wondered what would happen. She was in the transitional state between stages of AD, and that can be the emotionally wrenching for all involved. Most of the time I could comfort her, and she would relax. But I couldn't be with her all the time. In addition, the sibling antagonism was steady, and court was approaching; and I was protecting Mother from knowledge of that matter. I had to work with the homecare agency and the doctor, monitor the supplementary home aides, etc. It was simply overwhelming for one person. The sibling matter may have been the hardest of all.

If she thought clearly and could have understood the problem, Mother would have said, "I see, Heydon. This is too hard. We have to come up with a new solution." She was the most considerate of people and didn't want to be a burden to anyone. I was reminded of what she had said about my decision to stay and take care of her—"I don't want you to change your whole life just for me." She truly meant that.

I have seen a number of elderly people who don't hesitate to ask their offspring to take care of them in the needy years, asking them directly or indirectly. A person can understand their desperation at that time. However, Bernice was not in that group. Also, I know of offspring who dump their elderly parents in a nursing home prematurely, for the adult children's convenience. Dumping for convenience or monetary gain is not only the wrong thing to do morally, it's also very expensive for the government to subsidize an unnecessary resident at a nursing home.

*****

At home, Mother's anguish could be followed a little later by laughter at watching an old TV comedy which tickled her. The painful reactions were often followed by bouts of happiness. Severe confusion could be followed by clarity. The AD patient can go in and out of these states and not remember what they felt five minutes earlier. That's one reason it's hard to take certain definitive actions; nothing is black and white; two steps back, one step forward.

The family caregiver can be carried along on this emotional rollercoaster endlessly until it seems as though he or she is in a madhouse. I stress "family caregiver" here because the professional caregiver can automatically be more detached; they go to a residence or facility, put in their shift, and then go home. However, since Mother and I were at home and both sensitive people and tied in to each other's well-being, it was especially hard for me. When she felt pain, I felt pain; so, I wanted to do everything possible to stop that anguish, for her sake as well as mine.

When Bernice started having an episode while I was in another room, the aide would call me. My first thought was to comfort Mother and try to alleviate the distress that way. Most often that worked. In trying to comfort her, I would tell her that her confusion and fears were a result of the disease she had; further, that I was here with her and wouldn't let anything bad happen to her. Sometimes the comfort was just a matter of holding her.

If comforting didn't work, I tried to distract her with what was going on outside, or take her for a walk, or a trip to the garden if it was spring, summer or fall, or to offer her some other pleasant treat. At those times it was like dealing with your very small child—a child who looks to you for security and sustenance, and to "make the pain go away." When I was in such pain as a young child and turned to her for help, she was always there. Now, our roles had exactly reversed. All I could really do was to hold and comfort her, and assure her that we would get through this.

The aides were a help. I couldn't have kept Mother home that long without them. It just bothered me that Medicare and other health insurance would not assist with that most necessary and valid medical expense—a small expense compared to the exorbitant cost of nursing homes.

NH #2

On June 17, 1995, I went into Mother's bedroom and found her on the floor. She had fallen but didn't seem to be hurt. However, as I helped her up, she did feel pain when she tried to walk. I called for an ambulance, and she was taken to the emergency room. She didn't have any breaks, and the diagnosis was bursitis—inflammation of the joints.

Her primary care physician recommended convalescence and therapy again, so I was back searching for another nursing home. My first choice from the previous search had an opening, so we went through admissions again. This was a new, modern facility, and everything looked right.

Dejectedly, I walked with Mother to her two-person room, trying to be upbeat about the doctor's orders for staying here awhile. She didn't complain and was silent as we walked into her new quarters. In the bed closest to the door was a sturdy, big-boned woman who was staring at the wall in front of her. I said hello and introduced myself and Mother. This woman kept staring at the wall and didn't reply. I was caught up in our drama for the moment so I didn't think about the woman's silence. Then, while still staring at the wall, she said, "I'll tell you what. If you don't cut it out, I'll cut your goddamn hand off and throw it in to the pigs!" That got my attention. "Excuse me," I said. "What did you say?" With her eyes still fixed on the wall, she said, "I'm not kidding, dammit! I'll cut it off and throw it to the pigs!" She seemed pretty close to active violence. She must have been off in one of her life's traumatic moments.

That was enough for me. No way in the world could my mother be put in a room like that. Bernice was a petite, gentle lady who was already having trouble with the new order of staying in this facility, or any facility. I went to the office and said that wouldn't do. They made other arrangements and opened up a bed in a more peaceful room. Later on, I figured that Bernice's first assigned roommate may have been one of the mental patients being placed in area nursing homes since the central Indiana mental hospital had been closed down.

Once Bernice was set up in the room, I went to the dining area with her to find out where she would be sitting and then stayed with her for the meal. The dining room was very large and loud with so many people in it. In various areas of the room were about five or six residents acting out with loud moans and trying to stand up and leave. I looked at Bernice and saw her wincing at the shock of all that chaos. On my way out of the building that day, I spoke with the Administrator about the dining room condition. Before long, they took the very troubled and overactive people out of the main dining area and fed them in an adjoining room.

Every day Mother asked me to take her home. Softly and in a pleading voice, she would say, "Please take me home." Every day I would reply that we had to wait until the doctor said it was okay. She seemed to accept that, at least for five minutes until she would ask me again. It was so hard, so painful for both of us.

One day I went in, and I thought her request was going to break my heart. She was softly pleading, "Please take me home. If you could just find a little space for me, I promise I won't be any trouble. I promise." She even used her thumb and index finger to measure how small a space she needed. I left the facility and the tears started to fall. It was the most poignant scene I can remember. She spoke like a little girl who thought herself abandoned, perhaps for doing something wrong though she couldn't remember doing anything wrong. She had tearfully repeated herself a couple of times with "I promise I won't be any trouble. I promise. I promise."

Here was this true lady—my mother, a fully gentle soul, the closest semblance to a Christian I have ever known, the person who had done more for me than anyone else in my life, a human always giving joy and love—this person was in her hour of need, and I couldn't fulfill her wish. This person who had never been any trouble to anyone, and who had helped everyone who crossed her path was promising not to be "any trouble." This sweet invalid just wanted to be in the comfort and warmth and love of her own home, and I couldn't provide that with the medical rules that controlled us; and Mother couldn't understand those controls anymore. She may have thought that I just didn't want to take her home, even after I had explained about the doctor's orders.

Her plea and condition brought to mind a state of total innocence and trust. It was the deep sadness of someone with whom you had experienced unconditional love and now felt that she was being consciously abandoned and couldn't comprehend why. Of course the inability to communicate any of this is what made it frustratingly painful for me. There was no answer to make her feel better. Even if I had come up with a plan to eliminate her sense of abandonment, she would have forgotten it within minutes after I told her. It was just another example of the perpetual suffering that can afflict an Alzheimer's patient.

That night I went home and soaked in a hot tub with Epsom salts. I thought about the day, and it was so sad. I felt a despair that's hard to describe. My mother was suffering emotionally, and I didn't know how to stop that. I silently prayed for help in understanding all of this. I tried to relax and digest all the conditions and components that made up this chaotic situation.

After a little while, a smile started to spread across my face, and I said out loud, "You're coming home, Mother. You're coming home!" I laughed out loud and slapped the water time and again. Then I smiled my way to sleep, knowing that the next morning I would find a way to make it happen.

Mother entrusted me to be her Health Care Representative with her doctor's agreement, and it was time again to act in her interest. I contacted the home health care agency I had used before. We hadn't needed any aides for the past six weeks, since Mother had been in NH #2. The owner came by to arrange the aides' schedule with me and to make a contract. The basic support devices needed were already installed, still in place from when I brought Mother home from NH #1— stabilizing bars around the toilet, one bar for the wall side of the tub, and a shower hose to bathe more easily. As with Mother's previous nursing home release, the outside aides would take a twelve-hour shift,

and I would cover the other twelve hours. Once everything was final-
ized, I spoke with Bernice's doctor and told him of the preparations and
resources for her home care. The doctor agreed to recommend her release, and we were set to leave. It took about a week to get everything
arranged.

What a great day it was when I brought her home—August 9,
1995. She and I were both tickled to death. Some of the other nursing
home residents couldn't believe that one of their own was going home.
Residence in the "unskilled area" of a nursing home is usually a death
sentence—once you're in, you can plan to die there or at the hospital.

Some residents stared with mouths open, as though to ask,
"Why does she get to go home?" A couple of others smiled with understanding, as they had tapped into our well of joy. A couple of the staff
members were also surprised to see that Mother was getting a reprieve.
It was a sight they didn't see too often. And, I'm sure the administration
didn't want to lose a gentle, cooperative patient like Bernice.

It was incredibly wonderful. I wrote a short article about the
experience of bringing her home. It was printed in the *Indianapolis Star*
March 23, 1996. I'm reprinting it below as it appeared then. The *Star*
added the title. It read:

Alzheimer's can't steal their happiness

Joy is a special feeling. It may not be bliss, but neither is anything else in this world.

When joy is really running through you, it's like having Tupelo
honey in your veins and it makes you just shiver with comfort.

The best joy I ever felt was the day I finished service and got
out of the Army. A surge of freedom drove my mind and body in a rising crescendo from the second I awoke and dressed in Army green, until
late that night, when my head hit my home pillow and I was no longer a
soldier. I spent the day giggling in emotion, all smiles, bubbles probably
flying from my lips. I was alive; I was home; and I was free. That was 26
years ago.

Nine months ago, I went through my second greatest joy—I
brought my mother, Bernice Buchanan, home from the nursing home
for the last time of her life. Home to live—not for a day out or a family
dinner in, but home to sleep in her own bed, covered by her own quilt

and surrounded by her own personal things, not to mention the nourishment of close family love.

She was so happy she couldn't contain herself. Even though dementia had taken a good portion of her short-term memory, she was ecstatic.

She rushed me to get her out of the building, into the truck, and on our way home. She was laughing and crying, and I felt like her savior.

The joy pumped me up into the clouds, as I confirmed to myself, "This system's not taking my mother. Not while I can make a difference."

The drive home was more of the same. Our happiness kept rising. A lively and loving camaraderie was reborn, taken to a new level.

The conversation was limited to sentences of jubilation with the bonded "we," "us" and "our," while "I" or "me" rarely came up.

We were like Butch and Sundance or any single pair who had left captivity and were heading home. All was right with the world.

When we arrived home, Mother was quiet for a moment but still all smiles. Going inside the townhouse, she walked into every room and then said with some satisfaction, "It all looks the same."

We sat in the living room, and she slowly settled into her favorite chair.

As though stoking the fire, I asked her, "Are you happy to be home?"

Her smile then changed to a giggle as she said, "You bet I am!" Her face returned a smile as she took a couple of breaths and her eyes began to close. That was it; she was asleep, peacefully composed in her chair.

I felt wonderful. The day had been so rewarding, and there would be more—more days of good food, love, warmth and comfort.

Still, I knew there would probably come a day when I couldn't keep her at home any longer, when it would be beyond my capacity to do the million and one things necessary in caring for a person with Alzheimer's. Hopefully, her mind would be far enough gone at that point.

But that was not today. Today, we were the victors. Mother got her greatest wish. And I had the opportunity to return a favor for the person who had done more for me in life than anyone else. [end of article]

Patient Frustrations at Home and Nursing Home

One of the many difficult areas of AD for caregivers and patients to deal with is the coming and going of the patient's personal orientation and subsequent emotional reaction. Patients may or may not know where they are at any given time. This knowledge can be based on a number of things (e.g., their physical condition at the time, the room environment with or without familiar objects around, knowing or not knowing the people around them).

When Mother and I were together at home, she was not often in anguish since she knew me and knew that I was there to take care of her. Also, she was in familiar surroundings with the antiques and other collectibles she and Dad had gathered over many years. Further, she had lived in the townhouse for fifteen years, so she knew the space quite well.

As an example of this, I refer back to NH #1 where some of my siblings wanted her to stay. Bernice was very confused and downhearted in NH #1. Summarizing the therapist's notes from that period illustrates two important points: 1) She wanted very much to come home. ("I want to go home now," she kept telling the speech therapist.) 2) She was more comfortable and capable at home than in the nursing home. ("Pt. seemed comfortable at home, more relaxed & less confused. Able to verbalize & point out living areas, e.g., kitchen, dining room, living room, bedroom, bathroom, television.")

Sometimes when offspring put their parents in a nursing home, the adult children feel it's "for their own good." Assuming the offspring have nothing to gain from such a placement, maybe that's true if the elderly are a threat to others (e.g., won't stop driving, smoking in bed, etc.). However, I can't help but feel that forcing people into a nursing home—or at least before their time—is somewhat akin to the practice of putting animals in cages at the zoo. Imagine trapping an animal in its natural habitat and telling it, "We're going to put you in a cage at the zoo for the rest of your life. You'll like it. You'll have your own urine-soaked, concrete floor to pace back and forth on...pace endlessly in frustration...have people stare at you. We'll even hose you down. Plus we'll have three square meals a day for you. Then, if we feel like it, we'll come by and visit you sometime. Don't you feel fortunate? Isn't this your lucky day?" The analogy's not too far off when elderly, healthy people are forced into a facility against their will. There should be other choices. I will discuss this further in the final chapter.

A friend of mine worked as an ambulance driver while attending college. Among his passengers were some elderly patients who were going from the hospital to a nursing home; only those patients didn't know they were being carried to such a facility. They had been committed there by their loved ones without being told by anyone; and when they found themselves being dropped at the nursing home, they were really angry. My friend had heard some choice phrases that the elderly patients used for those family members who had secretly had them transferred there.

I'm reminded of the bumper sticker I saw six or seven years ago. It read, "Be nice to your kids. They'll be choosing your nursing home." The sticker may have been considered a joke, but as we now see, there's a bunch of truth in it.

NH #3

On September 18, 1995, I took my mother to a nursing home where I knew she would be for the rest of her natural life. It was certainly one of the hardest things I've ever done; and yet there was a measure of relief as I was totally exhausted at that point. I drove home from the facility and slept as if in a coma. I don't remember feeling guilty, for I knew that I had done everything possible to fulfill my promise to her. Actually I did fulfill my promise because I had promised to do my best, never ruling out a nursing home as a last resort.

Fortunately, her condition had then degenerated to the point where she just couldn't put it all together. She knew she was in a medical facility, but she didn't know that it was a nursing home. So, her heart didn't get broken by the feeling of being abandoned. I was grateful to God for the spiritual help to last until that point. Since Bernice walked in the Grace of God during her whole life, I didn't really believe she would be forsaken to a broken heart. She had already suffered enough.

Last year, I reviewed her medical records from that period at her primary care physician's office in order to make some notes. Her doctor had written in June—three months before she entered the nursing home—that I told him I didn't know if I could do this much longer.

Summer, 1995, NH #2, a brief stay
before our joyous escape (details in chapter nine).
Bernice, Nancy, and Heydon—the three musketeers

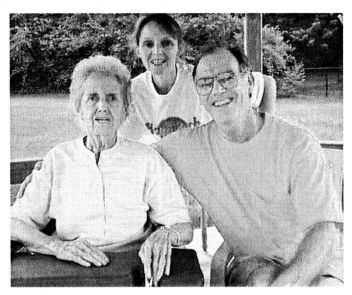

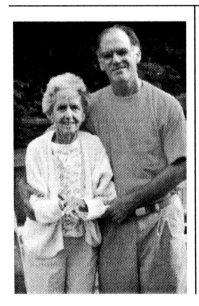

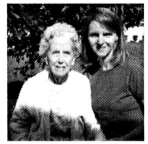

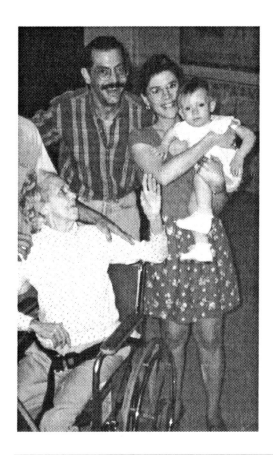

NH #3, 1996,
Visitors from afar—
Bernice's grandson
(Danny), his wife
(Lynn), and
great-granddaughter
(Caitlyn) come
by to visit.

Caitlyn
introduces
herself.

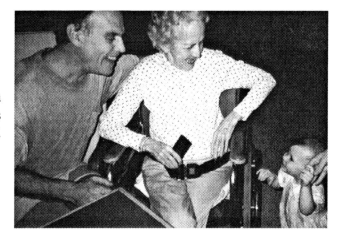

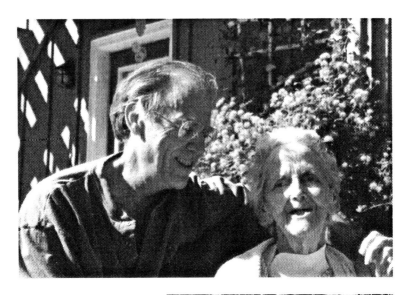

Summer, 1996,
Mother spending
the day with Nancy
and me at our home.
Alzheimer's couldn't
steal her smile.

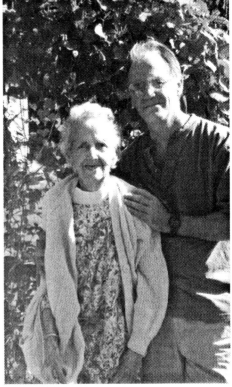

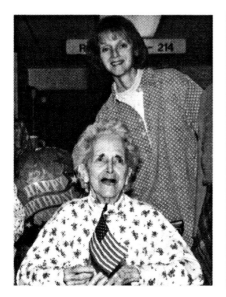
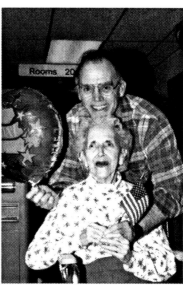

April 12, 1997, Bernice's 84th Birthday party
Spending the day with Nancy, Heydon, and other friends.

April 12, 1917, Bernice's 4th Birthday party
Another group of friends celebrate her life.
Bernice, front row, left.

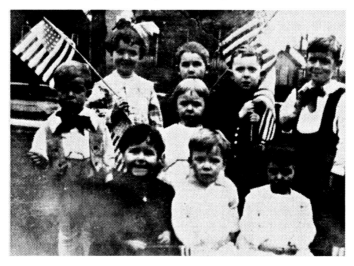

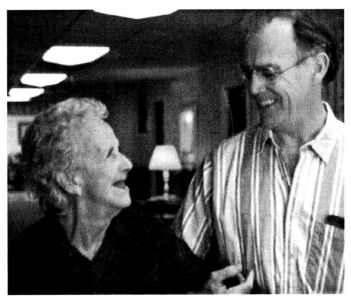

Thanksgiving, 1997
We all spent the day giving thanks
for having each other.

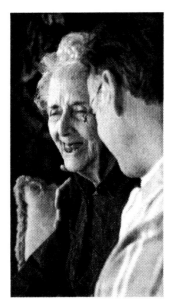

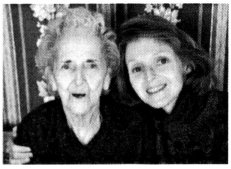

Innocence— wonder above
and giggles to the left.

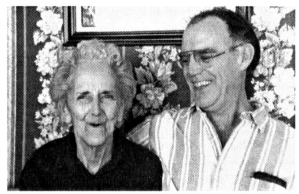

Two old friends sharing some joy.

A pause in the joy of being together. Possibly a meditation on the past, present, and future— as though to ponder, "We've been through so much to arrive at this point. What lies ahead of us?"

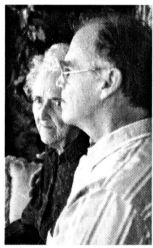

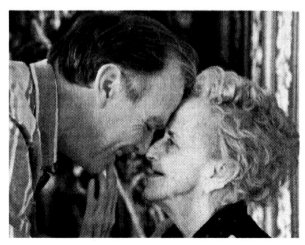

My favorite photo of the period— laugh lines in communion.

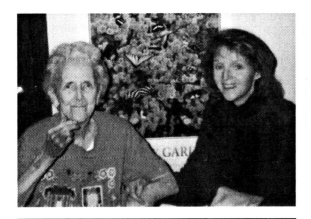

1998
Butterfly poster
behind Bernice
and Nancy.

1999

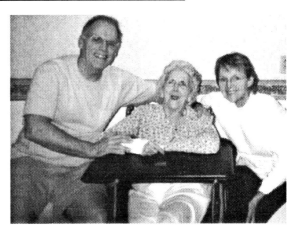

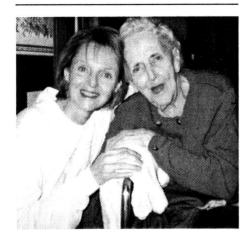

2000

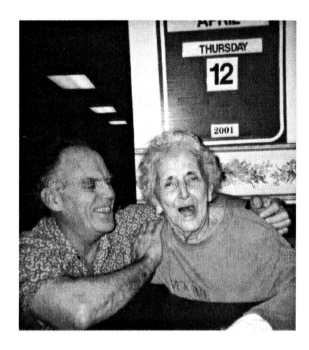

88th birthday
April 12th, 2001
Left and below

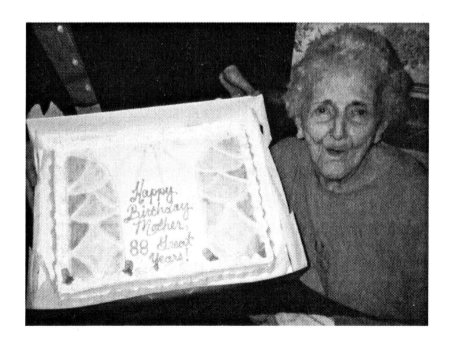

I had forgotten, or blocked out, that statement to him. However, Mother and I made it through, and it worked out.

I thought my responsibilities would diminish a great deal when she entered the nursing home, but that didn't turn out to be the case. It didn't take long to learn that the best thing you can do for your loved one in a nursing home is to maintain a presence.

Mother was still asking me every day to take her home. That continued for a long time. I told her that we had to wait for the doctor's okay before we could leave. That was true; however, I wasn't about to approach a doctor on the matter because I was beyond my capacity to handle home care any more. Another reason I gave for not taking her home was that I was on my way to work. This was true as I had gotten a job as a technical writer within months after I took Mother to the nursing home. Her reply to the "work excuse" was, "Oh good, then you can drop me off on the way." "No," I told her, "I have to go in the other direction." That was true also.

At one point I noticed that her request for me to take her home came at the end of my visit, when I said I had to be leaving. To avoid that trigger, I sometimes just mentioned I had to go the bathroom and then went home from there. Since her short-term memory was virtually non-existent at that point, she would soon forget when I was out of sight. I was able to stay honest in my answers, but they were evasive. Due to her inability to understand, I couldn't give a complete reply without it being misunderstood and subsequently hurting her more. Sometimes it was a challenge to keep my conscience clear and keep her balanced as well. I was able to do it, but it meant giving her partial answers at times.

Self-Attempts To Go Home

Mother's attempts to leave NH #3 and go home didn't just stop with her requests for me to take her home. She became a "roamer"; she would roam the halls and look for a door to release her into the outside world. The doors were locked, and also she had an ankle alarm which would go off if she slipped through a door as someone else was coming in.

There were handrails along the walls to help residents stabilize themselves as they walked. Even so, long-term residents eventually lost their balance and took a fall, sometimes getting banged up and very bruised. I saw a few residents who had fallen down face first and they looked like one solid bruise.

Within eighteen months Mother was spending most of her time in a wheelchair. That didn't stop, nor even slow down, her attempts to escape. On the contrary, she increased her speed a great deal over walking. She would wheel herself through the halls from one end to another looking for a door that was unlocked. She did this endlessly in her attempt to come home.

Her frail little hands and paper-thin skin were getting bruises and scratches quite easily from the rush to turn the chair's wheels. In order to protect her hands and skin, we put on some gloves without fingers and then a side bar to limit her access to the wheels.

That didn't stop her. She switched to using her legs and feet. She would paddle those feet so fast that people couldn't believe it when she passed them by in her wheelchair. The staff called her "Speedy." A wizened little lady of a hundred pounds with a determined look and her head bent forward as if to gain that tiny extra bit of momentum. You could tell that she was a lady with a mission. She kept on her endless search for a way out.

The escape attempts probably went on for a few years. When I was with her, she didn't try to escape. She was very relaxed and must have felt that she was at home. We were always comfortable with each other without exception. We had developed a great friendship during our caregiving process, and we shared a lot of love.

Her oldest friend came to visit her once in the nursing home. However, after a minute, Mother scooted off on her mission as Selma was to tell me later. Selma said, "Heydon, I just couldn't go back."

Selma was a few years younger than Mother, but her mind was sharp as could be. Her body would go before her mind. I believe that she—like so many people—was very uncomfortable being around AD patients. Also, the nursing home was not too far away in her future, so that may have been hard to face. Selma was an interesting woman. Raised on a farm in a small town in southern Indiana, she had moved to Indianapolis and become a nurse. She spoke slowly, but I could tell her mind was moving about three times as fast as she spoke…probably strategizing. I never heard her speak with emotion nor give any compliments; she spoke in a deadpan manner—somnolent. She and Mother seemed an odd pair, but they had gone to garage sales together for about thirty years. Also, with their husbands, they had garden plots behind Selma's church.

Selma moved away from Indy a little before Mother passed away. She called to check on Mother's condition, and I told her of the passing and funeral. That's when Selma told me about her trip to the nursing home and inability to go back another time. Perhaps in accord with her own limitations, Selma said, "I just don't understand how you were able to commit and take care of her for so long."

"Well," I started, "concerning my commitment, it was because she was such a special person—someone who had done a lot for me and others, and I loved her a great deal." Selma knew Mother well and would understand that. "Beyond that, I believe that the Grace of God helped us through."

"Well," she replied, "in my mind, you are two very special people."

"Thank you," I said, not knowing what else to say. I was in some shock. Hearing that from the ever-cautious Selma was like getting the Medal of Honor. As I mentioned before, nice words to the caregiver can go a long way.

That was the last conversation Selma and I had. She passed away last year in a nursing facility about two hundred miles south of Indy. Her body was brought here for burial, and I attended a memorial for her at her church. She and her husband are buried in the same cemetery as Mother and Dad.

Legal Problem

Within a few months after Mother's entry into the nursing home, her court-appointed financial guardian—a local lawyer from the court's available list— withdrew from Mother's case since there was no more money in her estate. Subsequently, my role changed from personal guardian to full guardian—a technicality since my responsibility was still for Mother's health and well-being. She no longer had outside bills or assets so the need for a financial guardian became a moot point.

Eighteen months after I became full guardian, I was at a quarterly care plan meeting and encountered an unexpected problem. We had finished reviewing Mother's condition and the proposed treatment plan for the next three months when a new issue came up. As I was standing to leave, the activities representative asked me, "How do you like Bernice's new clothes?"

"What new clothes?" I asked back.

The crux of the matter was that Mother's former financial guardian had recently authorized a $500 expenditure from her nursing home personal account. A combination of administrative errors led to that happening, starting with the fact that the nursing home had not properly filed the change of financial guardian from eighteen months earlier. So, the attorney shouldn't have been called for any authorization expenditure; he had no part in Bernice's life. I was not so upset with the activities person (a gentle and helpful lady)—though the nursing home had made the initial mistake—but I wanted a copy of that authorization. She couldn't find it in the records and called the attorney to get a copy from him, mentioning that I was upset about the matter. It seemed that he hadn't saved a copy either. As reported to me, the attorney replied to the activities person, "If Heydon has a problem with it, tell him to call me." Well, of course, as Mother's full guardian, I had a problem with it—unauthorized spending from her nursing home account. Since he had been court-appointed and charging $125 an hour (1996 rate)—he should have known what he was doing. He didn't even remember that Mother wasn't his client anymore, and hadn't been for eighteen months since he had filed his guardianship release with the state declaring that she had no more money in her account. His recent unauthorized spending reminded me of our first consultation with him—he took so many phone calls I wondered if he could stay on track with our case, considering all those interruptions. I also wondered if he could remember all of those clients, and I was now finding out that he couldn't.

No, I sure didn't have time to straighten that attorney out. I thought that should be up to his peers—his law partners and the bar association. That would be the most meaningful lesson for him. On November 5, 1997, I wrote a note concerning the incident to the Disciplinary Commission of the Supreme Court in Indiana. The Commission acknowledged receipt and said they would be in touch. Two and a half months later, they replied with the following: "This matter was investigated by the Grievance Committee of the Indianapolis Bar Association. After reviewing the complaint and studying the results of the investigation, we have determined that it does not raise a substantial question of misconduct that would warrant disciplinary action. Therefore, the complaint has been dismissed. Thank you for bringing this matter to the attention of the Disciplinary Commission. Sincerely, _____, Executive Secretary"

I believe the Grievance Committee chose their language carefully—"does not raise *a substantial question of misconduct* [my italics]." I didn't consider it an action of substantial misconduct either. I didn't think it was malicious or larcenous. I simply believed it was sloppy and incompetent. I would imagine that the committee had a few private words for the attorney though. I imagine his partners had a few words for him as well. Not long after this, his firm sent a check for $500 to Mother's nursing home account with the explanation that when the attorney had closed out his financial guardianship eighteen months earlier and said there was no money left in Mother's account, there had actually been an active account with $500 in it; funny that it was just the amount that he had improperly authorized. I guess they were afraid of being sued. If that attorney had been halfway decent with me previously instead of indifferent and somewhat arrogant, I probably would have just dropped the matter. However, I believe he'll pay more attention now to the business at hand and act in a professional manner; and his subsequent clients should benefit by my action. Primary caregivers/health care representatives/guardians need to share with other current or future caregivers what we've learned in the process and the system.

I mention the above case because it illustrates just one more detail that the caregiver/guardian has to keep an eye on. There are a million and one facets of the patient's care and affairs to monitor, and never enough time to complete everything. One relevant book title about Alzheimer's disease says it all—*The 36-Hour Day.*[1]

Staff and Daily Care

Not long after Mother's entry into NH #3, I noticed a change in the quality of patient service. The facility seemed to be sliding downward. One of the principal problems was that too many permanent staff were calling in sick on weekends. As a result, replacements were brought in from temporary (temp) agencies. That brought its own set of problems: 1) temp CNAs and nurses not knowing the patients; 2) a higher rate of theft of patient's personal items; 3) some medications disappear-ing from the medicine cart; 4) a diminished sense of responsibility to the patients by the some of the temps since they would be there for such a brief period. Of course, the problem of theft does not apply to all temps nor is it limited to temps.

A further problem is that temporary agencies charge a great deal of money for the service, and that money could be used in other areas of the facility to improve care. Beyond that, temps usually make a higher wage than permanent staff, and that causes resentment among the per-manent, responsible staff who have shown up on the weekends instead of calling in sick.

Another problem was the abnormal turnover of Administrators and DONs. Those are the two major positions in a nursing home and changing the person in either position can change the whole character of service and quality in the facility.

Family Council

Another resident's son and I worked to organize other resident family members to form a Family Council. The purpose of this group was to work with the administration of the facility, as well as the corpo-rate owners of the nursing home, in order to improve quality and consis-tency of care. This included getting substantial raises for the CNAs who were making below average wages and had a very high turnover rate which was not good for the facility or the residents.

This Family Council work took a lot of time. Since I was already working full-time at my regular job of technical writing, plus overtime, plus substantial commuting time, and then visiting Mother at night, I was stretched very thin.

It was during this period that we five offspring received the $10,000 each from Mother's trust—money which had been set aside some years earlier. As mentioned previously, I still felt this was Mother's money; further, the fairest and best use of it would be to benefit Mother in some way. I decided what would help her most was for me to spend more time on the problems at the nursing home—problems that I will detail below. This translated to more time working on the Family Coun-cil to obtain improved care for her and the other residents. So, I resigned from my regular job and concentrated on trying to fix the short-comings at the facility.

To augment my inheritance, I signed up to be a substitute teacher in the local school system. I usually did that a few days a week to get some additional income. Also, schools let out early enough in the day that I could get a workout/aerobics class in before going to the nursing home in the evening.

Sometimes I would reflect on how rich in exposure and interaction my daily life was. During the day, I was working with kids from five to eighteen. In late afternoon, I worked out at the gym with people from eighteen to sixty-five. In the evening, I worked with, and for, people who were sixty-five to ninety. A regular weekday in my life often involved working and socializing with people from five to ninety. I was an active part of lives that represented the full age spectrum on all those days.

*****

There was now more time to work on the agenda of the Family Council. We were making progress. Most importantly, the corporate owners of the nursing home were beginning to listen seriously to our concerns. We represented about thirty resident families, and the corporation definitely didn't want to lose the large amount of money we represented; that is, if we decided to take our residents out of their facility. Since this was a profit-making institution, the corporate representative was very interested in keeping that large block of customers.

My friend and I invested a lot of time in the Family Council. Part of the work was on organizing the agenda and notifying family members to join us; part was on developing a new schedule with weekend workers, so it would eliminate all of the sick call-ins on the weekend. There would be weekday workers and weekend workers—everyone would be happy. Another big concern was the high turnover of Administrators and DONs. These two facility leaders are the most influential positions in a nursing home, and their attitudes and practices set the tenor of an institution. The staff was interested in the council as well since we had their interests at heart and wanted to work hand-in-hand with them for the betterment of all. Everyone seemed enthusiastic about the proposed weekday/weekend work schedule, but the Administrators didn't really follow up. I had invested a lot of time in working out the details of this schedule and had charted it all out. Then, we were sort of shined on concerning this issue.

There were two principal improvements resulting from the Family Council's work, and both were very important. First, we were instrumental in getting raises for the CNAs which lowered their attrition rate. Second, we were able to get a new Administrator and DON—the two key positions in a nursing home. These two new leaders were both capable and conscientious, and a great improvement over the prior administration which operated from a defensive posture instead of a proactive and cooperative position.

When I first brought Mother to NH #3, it was a good facility to the best of my knowledge. Actually, I had been touring another facility two blocks away at the time. Speaking with a nurse privately, I asked, "Would you bring your Mother to this facility?" She replied, "No."

"Where would you take her?" I continued.

"Right down this street is a better facility [NH #3]," she answered.

So I toured the recommended facility. Then, having compared NH #3 and the other facilities I had considered earlier, I chose NH #3.

While NH #3 was pretty good at that time, it started going downhill shortly afterward. I believe there were eight different Administrators and DONs in a two-year period. That's a sign that something is very wrong. That's when we on the Family Council stepped in. As a result, I believe my portion of the inheritance was well-spent and for Bernice's benefit—our Family Council had done its job, and I was also able to spend a lot more time with Mother which meant a great deal to her.

Nursing Home Staff

If you are going to be involved in your loved one's care at a facility, then you need to know the staff. Introduce yourself to at least one person from each department; and ask what they do, as well as asking what you can do to help in their service to your family member. Working together is the key to everything with open communication as much as possible.

Administrator—This is the top position at the nursing home—the person who oversees the whole operation. If you have an Administrator with an "us vs. them" (staff vs. resident families) attitude, then you could have a serious problem in getting the best care for your loved one; that is, with that attitude, the Administrator is reluctant to share information with the "customers."

DON (Director of Nursing)—The #2 position at a nursing home in terms of overall influence. The DON is in charge of all hands-on patient care. That includes supervision of the nurses (RN & LPN), CNAs (Certified Nursing Assistants), and QMAs (Qualified Medication Aides). The DON should be visible in the building and not always closed away in his or her office. Also, the DON should practice hands-on patient care and teach by example.

Social Worker—This position coordinates patient entry into the nursing home—from the hospital as well as home—and helps resident families in a variety of socialization issues (e.g., coordination of roommates and patient behavior issues).

Admissions Director—The most visible position for families seeking a facility for their loved one. This person is the facility's principal liaison to the outside world and conducts tours for prospective clients/customers, as well as answers all questions about requirements for placement and life in the facility.

Accountant/Bookkeeper—The person handling all payments to NH for service—from private pay, insurance, Medicare, and Medicaid sources. Also makes payments to suppliers. Further, maintains patient personal accounts—the small accounts patients have to pay for hair care, cable TV, clothing, and whatever else they wish to purchase.

CNAs (Certified Nursing Assistants)—If not the most important position with regard to hands-on patient care, it is the hardest physically. These people have to lift and turn the patients, change personal undergarments, dress patients, feed, and bathe them. Resident family members should share with the CNAs as much patient personal information/needs as possible to get the most efficient care for their loved ones.

QMAs (Qualified Medication Aides)—These employees distribute medications to patients.

RNs (Registered Nurses)—These nurses are only required to be on duty on the Medicare/skilled care unit.

LPNs (Licensed Practical Nurses)—These nurses manage the unskilled care unit which principally treats long-term dementia patients and some stroke victims and others.

Activities Director—This person schedules group activities as well as activities tailored to individual needs. Resident families should consult with her or him to work on a plan suited to the loved one's needs.

Maintenance—These employees—men in my experience—handle a variety of building maintenance functions, to include electrical and small-scale construction. Also, they make sure the building is compliant with all building construction codes and safety codes. Further, they can make minor alterations in the patient's room to make life more pleasant and functional (e.g., hanging pictures, putting up a TV stand, mounting a stand for a birdfeeder outside the patient's window).

Housecleaning—These employees keep the building clean—patient's rooms, hallways, restrooms, etc. They seem to be more visible in the evening as they clean and buff the hallways when few other people are around.

Laundry—These employees are charged with cleaning a mountain of laundry. The washers and dryers seem to run constantly. Sheets, blankets, clothing, et al are always coming or going. It is important to have your loved one's clothing marked with an indelible pen so the clothing will be returned to him or her; if clothing is not marked, you will often see patients wearing clothing that is not theirs. Also, you should be careful with the type of material in patient's clothing; it could shrink a great deal in those high-heat dryers. You always have the option of taking some or all of patient's clothing home to clean there.

Dietary/Kitchen—Everyone involved in food preparation. The supervisor is the good person to speak with concerning your loved one's diet (e.g., salt/no salt, sugar/no sugar, milk/no milk, regular texture/ pureed, sipper cup, etc.).

Working with Nursing Home Staff

Every patient's family wants their loved one to have the best care possible. To achieve this, family members need to do at least several things.

The most important thing you can do for your loved one in a nursing home is to maintain a presence there. Keep your eyes open for how your family member and others are being treated in every way. Many personnel will be conscientious enough to do their best whether you are around or not. Others may not be so diligent, and your being there could make a big difference in how well your loved one is cared for.

Work with staff to let them know as much as possible about your family member's interests, as well as his or her likes and dislikes. Also, tell the staff of the patient's abilities, former occupation, hobbies, etc. The more information staff members have about the patient, the better they can construct an effective care plan.

To my knowledge, no patient wants to be in a nursing home, so it can be quite a challenge to design a constructive and effective daily plan of action. Think of the facility's staff as your partners in designing a happy and healthy daily life for your loved one.

Staff Performance—The Good and The Bad

Similar to any business, the staff of a nursing home is composed of conscientious and effective employees, as well as those who don't harmonize well. Hopefully, those who shouldn't be there will be weeded out. While the staff may monitor new employees for a breaking-in period, residents' families should also watch new hands-on employees to see that loved ones are receiving proper care. For that matter, family members should monitor all of their loved one's care to make sure the treatment meets the patient's needs.

Almost 95% of my nursing home experience as a family member was at NH #3, so I'll speak of the employees I knew and interacted with there. I've already mentioned the maintenance men above who did exceptionally good work and were always available to help residents and their family members make their living areas more pleasant. NH #3 was fortunate to have some very capable and personable men in that department. Phil, Jack and their staff were always helpful and pleasant.

The people who will spend the most time with your loved one, to include the most hands-on time, are the CNAs. They have a strenuous job, and those who do it well deserve more respect than they normally receive. They have perhaps the highest turnover rate of any profession in the facility.

The nurses that I interacted with daily were LPNs. Bernice was on the unskilled unit, the second floor of the building. No RN was required for that area. An RN was downstairs in the skilled care area and available on an emergency basis for the second floor. I knew some very good and dedicated nurses over the years. I made it a point to thank them for their work, acknowledge them to the DON and the Administrator, and write letters of recommendation for their personnel files, hoping that the letters would be considered when it was time for their salary review. I was closer to some of them than to some of my own siblings. We were part of each other's daily lives for years and years. I saw them have children and raise families, and we worked together to make the best possible situation for Mother and the other residents there.

I also knew some nurses who didn't last long because of one personal problem or another. I was sympathetic to their problems but didn't want them working with Bernice or other residents when their caregiving was compromised by external stresssors. The nurses' problems could range from marital strife to substance abuse to blatant disregard for patient welfare. One case in particular bothered me a lot. There was a nurse who lasted four months before being fired. While she appeared to be doing everything right in patient care, it was later exposed that she was callously and secretively doing some practices which would harm the patients. I'll name her Jane.

I went in to visit Mother one evening and noticed that Jane wasn't in. Then I learned from another nurse that Jane had been let go, but no other information was available. Eventually I learned the following. During the last two months of Jane's employment, there were a number of behavior problems among the residents: some were very aggressive toward other residents and staff; there were increased crying episodes, wandering, etc.; and the number of falls almost tripled. After trying various solutions to correct these problems and without positive results, the staff finally did a pill inventory. It turned out that Jane had not been giving some of the patients their medications but had still signed the medication sheet certifying that the meds. had been given. Worse yet, she had only withheld medications from the cognitively-impaired patients, those who couldn't express themselves, or wouldn't be listened to, especially if it was their word against Jane's. So, Jane was confronted; she didn't dispute the accusations; and she was then discharged.

The system following such discharge involves the forwarding of pertinent information to the Health Professions Bureau (HPB) who

then sends a recommendation to the Attorney General to see if that office wants to take further action (i.e., a license review), something to
protect consumers against this happening again with this person. In the
past, the Indianapolis HPB proved very lackadaisical in forwarding these
reports; also, the Attorney General had discretionary powers on follow
through or prosecution. The bottom line was that a lot of patient abuse
cases seemed to fall through the cracks. The abusive nurse could then
just walk down the street and get another job doing the same thing. I
couldn't let this case slide. I kept asking the facility Administrator to follow through and find out what action had been taken. For a trusted
medical professional to abuse cognitively-impaired patients like that was
something that bothered me terribly. I wrote a letter to Mother's doctor,
who was also the facility's medical director, and pressed the matter.
When I encountered him a week later, he didn't seem interested in pursuing further action. He said these things just happen sometimes in facilities and probably always would. I told him that I might go to the
newspaper with the case. He replied that that would just hurt the facility.
This doctor was released as medical director of NH #3 not long after
that. A review of patient medical records showed that he had not been
making the number of patient visits agreed upon in his contract. I had to
find that out through back channels as well.

       Although I was alone in my fervor to pursue this abusive nurse,
I did get cooperation from the Administrator to keep pressing this case
as he communicated with the Attorney General's office. Without his
cooperation, I would have gone to the newspaper. To greatly shorten
this story, I will say that Jane was summoned several times for a license
hearing, never showed up, and eventually—19 months later—her license
was suspended for three years. It was basically a one-man crusade, but I
got it done and subsequently that nurse was not able to abuse other dementia cases similarly for at least a few years. I could have just dropped
that case as everyone else was willing to do, but that was wrong. I mention this matter as just another one of those items that the caregiver has
to watch for continually.

       I should add a postscript to that case. After hearing the weak
response from Mother's doctor, I actually did go to the newspaper, to an
investigative reporter who had written much on the problems of nursing
homes in the Indianapolis area. When I told her about the problems

with this nurse and the Health Professions Bureau, she was understanding but said that she couldn't really comment because she herself was involved in an active investigation in that exact subject of improper nursing and the ineffective HPB. So, I worked on bringing the abusive NH #3 nurse to resolution while the reporter worked on the bigger picture of impaired nurses in the state and the ineffectual response of the HPB. Soon after Jane's case was finally handled properly, the reporter published her series of articles on the impaired nurses and the HPB. The State Attorney General had to get involved. The executive director of the Health Professions Bureau was quickly dismissed and the whole HPB organization was overhauled. That was just another side challenge during my caregiving years.

*****

As I said earlier, most of the staff are helpful and sincere in their work. Some are quite exceptional. I would advise residents' families to maintain a close relationship with the staff. Acknowledge them when they do well. Compliment them, bake them cookies, or however else you can pay tribute to the work they're doing. By working together, you'll be doing your best to assure your loved one's proper care.

Joyful Gifts and Coping Extras for the Nursing Home Patient

This portion is written primarily for the benefit of families who are new to the system. While it will illustrate my attempts to improve Mother's time at the nursing home, more importantly it may provide ideas or spin-off thoughts on how to make your loved one's stay as comfortable as possible.

The best gift that you can give your loved one or friend in a nursing home is to maintain a presence there as much as possible. There are two important reasons for that. First, just by being there and spending time with them, they know that you care; also, you can hold them, and give them hugs and kisses at a time in their lives when touch and affection are so important to the condition of their spirit.

Second, maintaining a presence at the nursing home is the best way to gauge the quality of service given to your loved one and the other residents. This is especially important for family members whose loved one has dementia, and can't tell you what treatment they did or didn't receive, or how they got a bruise or skin tear.

The monthly charge for life in a standard nursing home covers little more than room and board in terms of materials provided. There are other services included—activities, maintenance, laundry, bookkeeping, social services, etc.

However, when it comes to special items for residents, it is up to family members and friends to provide those. This includes anything small or large that you feel will make a difference in your loved one's life, something to ease the impersonal and uniform side of that existence. Beyond maintaining a presence at the nursing home, I tried to improve various facets of Bernice's life there with a series of comforts.

*****

Most residents have a television in their room, usually brought from home or purchased by a family member. They may also have a few pieces of furniture that had been part of their daily life at home. Beyond that, most families bring in clothing for their loved ones, as well as occasional special treats to eat—a birthday cake or Christmas cookies or some candy. Most of the family members won't be visiting very often though. According to one nurse at NH #3, only about ten to fifteen percent of the residents had a family member visiting them three or more times a week.

There are also residents who have no visitors and who receive nothing. These could be residents without family, or those whose family members just don't visit. A state guardian will legally represent the incompetent residents who have no family.

Each family or family member addresses this issue separately—that of making their relative/loved one feel as comfortable as possible in the situation. At first the trauma of placing and being placed in a nursing home take precedence over everything else. In the initial entry at the facility, families generally bring the personal home items/furniture that I mentioned earlier. In my case, I began considering extra comforts for Mother right after she had entered the home.

Chocolate, Church, and Similar Joys

As I remember, the first "extra" I brought to Mother was chocolates. Like so many millions of us, Mother found some comfort in the soothing power of chocolate. She always ate it in very small quantities like an "aficionado"—perhaps an after-dinner mint or a scoop of ice cream…eating silently and in contemplation until a smile would spread across her face.

At the facility, in the confusion of wondering where she was, my visits and the taste of chocolate helped to center her. She could have a respite from cares for a little while. And, I believe that she felt wherever I was, was home; for my part, even without dementia, I felt that wherever she was, was home.

As sparks of recognition began leaving her eyes during the course of the disease, I often wondered which of two words and concepts would leave Mother's recollection first—would it be "church" or "chocolate"? Both of those were lifelong institutions for her. I must say that chocolate eventually won out. In fairness, I should add that church was more important to her, but we couldn't go to church anymore, so she began to forget about it. On the other hand, I brought her chocolate at least a couple times a week, so that pleasure was regularly reinforced. I had taken Mother to church for a while after she entered the nursing home, but it became increasingly difficult as described earlier.

A curious thing happened whenever I brought Mother chocolates, and any other person was nearby; that is, within a large room where they may have been watching TV or interacting with other residents. I would bring her the chocolate and then offer the box for her to choose what she wanted. She would make an ever-so-slight shake of her head to say no. Then in an equally subtle move, her eyes would point in the direction of the other people, and her head would nod just a touch. The message was clear to me, "Offer the other people the chocolate before you give a piece to me." Knowing her character and personality, I was aware of the unspoken extension of that thought, "If you run out of chocolate before you get back to me, that's okay, I'll get a piece next time." That was her character through and through—always thoughtful of others first and very happily self-sacrificing. The other people in the room weren't even aware of us, but that didn't matter. Dementia was having a hard time changing that graciousness and was not successful until near the end of her life when she was far into final stage; at that point, it didn't destroy her gentility, but it became difficult for her to recognize other people being nearby.

The chocolates brought a problem that Mother couldn't possibly comprehend. I would gladly have brought enough chocolates for everyone and offered them first to others per her desire. However, this is something you don't do in a nursing home for various reasons. Most importantly, a number of those residents are diabetic, and the sugar would be unhealthy for them. Another reason is that the residents' families might not want them having such a treat for whatever reason. Mother couldn't comprehend these things. In her state of mind, she was no longer able to understand what diabetes was. But, manners and consideration for others are more deeply ingrained in a human than intellectual understanding; at least they were with Bernice.

Fortunately, after years passed, she was only able to focus on our interaction. Subsequently, she was able to enjoy the treats without feeling concern that the other nearby residents didn't have any. Before that, I would have to take her to her room or another separate area without people around where she could enjoy the chocolate without her concern about treating others first.

One note on the chocolates themselves—the criteria I used in choosing them were: 1) her favorites; 2) the texture; and 3) good quality. I generally stuck to buying her favorites—the thin chocolate wafers with peppermint centers. The texture had to be fairly soft since chewing was hard on her remaining teeth. For variety, I would bring her fudge and other specialties from a local fudge company.

Another sweet treat I brought her regularly was ice cream. It gave her much pleasure, and the quality was quite a step up from the standard fare at nursing homes. I learned to avoid flavors that had nuts and fruit in them because she would chew and chew until she had finally pulverized those solids; accordingly, it could take quite a while to get through a cup of ice cream. The chewing action, and the reason for chewing, are so deeply ingrained in us that they stay long after the mind has left.

On birthdays and some holidays, I brought a cake. That was always soft and easy to chew. Another addition that was easy on the teeth was soft cookies. Chocolate chip cookies were her favorite, and the chips melted easily without a chewing marathon.

Nutritious Treats

Moving toward the healthy and nutritious end of the pendulum, I made fresh fruit and vegetable juices for her. Having been juicing for several years, I had made her the juices at home and continued to make some to take to her at the nursing home. These juices had a high level of nutrients and enzymes, and I felt that they could only benefit her. Of course they had to taste good for her to drink them. Carrot juice was a favorite, and it was naturally sweet. Again, Mother was beyond any logic or understanding, so it was like feeding a baby.

The elderly have increasing difficulty in absorbing nutrients. Their immune systems are weaker as well, allowing winter cold and flu bugs to spread quickly. Since the older folks also tend to have little appetite and subsequently lose weight, it is an area that requires attention—an area that is also quite a challenge. I bought the best liquid vitamins I could find; they are absorbed more quickly and lose less of their potency than tablets or capsules. Then I would stir that blend into an appealing fruit juice and give it to Mother.

All nursing homes that I know of use supplemental liquid shakes—either commercial or house-version—for residents who need them for weight gain or nutrition. They are very high calorie, but I'm not sure about nutritive value. From my perspective as Bernice's guardian, I agreed to their use at times when her weight went way too low—due to a temporary illness and dehydration—and subsequently her doctor recommended the shakes. I was interested in augmenting the quality of her life but not quantity or longevity; good quality life will take care of longevity.

In the second year of Mother's stay at the nursing home, while the facility was on a downslide in overall quality of care, her weight dropped to 95 lbs., down about nine or ten pounds from her entry into the home about eighteen months earlier.

Bernice wouldn't always drink the shakes, so I had to think of another approach. When she wouldn't drink those, I made another drink for her using weight-gain powder—normally used by bodybuilders—which I bought at a health food store. For added sweetness, I would use maple syrup or honey. The maple syrup (grade B) is especially good nutritionally for the trace minerals it contains.

Coupling those drinks and the help of a newly-hired, capable and conscientious dietitian, Bernice's weight stabilized and then very slowly rose to top out around 100 lbs. Mother was five feet tall and appeared like a delicate, little bird.

Vitamin and Herbal Supplements

Another area of concern to me involved supplements that could make Bernice's life better. Vitamins and herbal supplements need to be approved by the patient's doctor. Once supplements are approved, the facility nurses should be made aware of their use by the resident. Actually, the nurses will probably administer them.

The first supplement I wanted Bernice to have was cranberry capsules. I had been using fresh cranberries in making fruit juices and believed in their value—not only for vitamin C, but also for keeping the urethra healthy and free of bacteria.

This last benefit is especially important in the nursing home setting and most especially for incontinent females there. The free movement of bacteria causes many of them in nursing homes to get urinary tract infections (UTIs). Also, some people are more susceptible than others. Over the years, Mother averaged between two and three of these a year at the nursing home. I wanted Bernice to be taking these cranberry capsules as a deterrent, although they never eliminated UTIs altogether. The doctor agreed and approved of their use.

My next request was for the use of time-released melatonin since AD patients have a mixed-up clock and often don't sleep well at night. The doctor okayed this suggestion as well, so I brought those along with the cranberry capsules for her use. The next item I requested approval for was gingko—an over-the-counter, "memory enhancing" herb. From what I had read, it seemed to help some people but not others. Here I was groping to stabilize the memory loss, since I didn't believe there was much chance to improve it. The doctor agreed to its use also.

We briefly tried a few other herbal recipes as well for relaxation. These were valerian root, "Rescue Remedy" (made of flowers), and ginseng (American roots which are known for providing relaxation). These were only done briefly, so I can't really comment accurately on their effectiveness. Ginseng especially has more of a cumulative effect, so it would have taken a lot of time to test that one more accurately.

All of the dietary supplements and tools for herbal relaxation were given in order to improve quality of life, not quantity. The whole concept was to increase comfort by minimizing physical, mental, and emotional suffering.

*****

During the course of her six plus years at the nursing home, there were a number of other additions I believed would improve her daily life. Part of my logic for the extras I brought in was that I would have wanted such things if I were in that state. However, I also knew Mother pretty well and our similarities in simple pleasures. Other items were chosen simply by intuition as her condition continued to decline, and her senses began to change in intensity.

There was no precedent to follow in choosing things. The staff did have some general recommendations (e.g., furniture or framed photos from home to give familiarity). However, they hadn't even imagined a lot of the things I brought in, and they were always pleasantly surprised to see these new innovations.

Pillows, Mattress, and Bed Linen

Whether ill or healthy, all people need good rest, and part of that is controlled by the equipment involved. As with other areas, I wanted to aid Mother's rest to maintain her health. I bought a few hi-tech, tempurpedic items: a three-inch mattress pad; a pillow; and a cushion for her wheelchair. The pad seemed to help, but was too wide for the bed and made changing the bed more difficult for the aides. The pillow didn't have the flexibility Mother was used to, so she couldn't adapt. The cushion for the wheelchair was very useful and molded to her form; it was quite comfortable and may well have helped avoid irritations on her bottom since she didn't have much body padding at that point.

For bed linen, I brought in some high-thread-count cotton which was very soft and comfortable. Two potential problems with this—the linens need to be identified with an indelible marker to avoid being misplaced, and the industrial dryers in a nursing home can shrink such sensitive fabrics. If I were doing this again, I would choose a fabric not subject to much shrinkage.

Lighting

I began to think of color in the room, and the effect it had on the residents. Choosing blue for its relaxing qualities, I brought in blue cellophane and wrapped two of the fluorescent lights in it. Those two could be turned on separately, so the choice was always available to use the blue ones or the conventional white light. The fluorescent bulbs didn't build up any heat, especially on the cellophane-covered portions, so there wasn't any fire hazard. This change did seem to help somewhat with Mother's relaxation once she was in bed. I would sit in the chair next to the bed and just talk with her. I definitely felt more relaxed with the blue color. To begin with, it was a softer feel. A light blue aura filled the room, and for a while we were transported away from the standard nursing home atmosphere. The staff noticed a different feeling in the room as well.

Clothing

Concerning clothing, I began by taking some of her favorite items—dress and casual. However, not long after, I learned about the need for simple clothing, such as light sweat suits. This is especially important when someone becomes incontinent or may drop food on her lap and require a change of clothes more often.

Some of the newer fabrics are a good choice for life at the nursing home. I bought some fleece tops that were very soft, comfortable, attractive, and easily taken off.

Shoes were another item to consider. Again, comfort soon became the most important factor. Although she had a couple pairs of dress shoes, Mother actually had more tennis shoes. Eventually I found some attractive shoes that were also very comfortable. By that time, Mother was confined to a wheelchair; she didn't need them for walking but even in the wheelchair there was a comfort to wearing them. And of course, comfortable socks were a necessary complement to the shoes.

We made sachet bags of lavender that I put in her clothing drawers. Bernice had actually made the attractive, pull-string bags, and it was one of the last sewing projects she had completed before those skills began to drift away. We had previously given some away as little Christmas gifts. At this point, I simply added the lavender and then took them in for her drawers.

Scents and Air Filter

Next was the matter of scents for the room. There isn't a steady smell in any decent nursing home as many people might imagine. However, the odor of incontinence does come up to some degree and must be dealt with. Sometimes the staff would use an air freshener after changing someone. I preferred a more natural, low-level, lingering scent.

At first, I bought some natural fragrances that could be sprayed in the room without being overwhelming. Then I moved to potpourris of various herbs. I thought lavender worked best since it's known to provide a sense of relaxation as well as being an air freshener.

Finally, I found a mini air freshener that plugged into the electrical outlet and dispersed a scent at a very low rate from an attached container of essence oil. The three-ounce container would last at least two months. This was the best choice for fragrance though it didn't become available until Mother's last two years.

On the subject of air quality, the next addition was a large HEPA air filter to eliminate the dust in the air. It was effective, as I found out when I cleaned the filter. Also, the steady hum of the motor probably helped lull Bernice to sleep.

Toiletries

Another consideration involves the toiletries that can make life at the facility a little more comfortable. Most necessary are the moisturizers. A drying atmosphere plus the advanced age of the residents makes their skin very vulnerable to drying and cracking. Mother's skin became almost translucent and as thin as paper. Some lotions may be used at the facilities, but again this practice is sporadic due to the ever-changing staff—the aides who usually apply lotion after a shower.

I brought in a combination of lotions and creams, each to be used depending on the condition of the skin. Sometimes I would leave them in her chest of drawers and tell the aides where they were. Also, I could apply the lotion during my visits. It was helpful to ID these bottles with Mother's name, as that made it less likely for them to get lost or taken. If it were an especially good therapeutic lotion, I would give it to the nurse who could put it with their supplies and bring it out as necessary. Again, this is a strategy to help avoid theft. I didn't want to store things in a cabinet at the nursing station because the aides might forget to use them. Still, some lotion bottles were taken, even when they were well-tagged, I came up with a new strategy. I made some little box labels with 14 point bold type caps which read: "WARNING: IF YOU TAKE THIS BOTTLE FROM BERNICE, YOU WILL HAVE BAD LUCK FOR THE REST OF YOUR LIFE." That was approaching morality from a different direction. Those labels were pretty effective. I don't remember any of those bottles being taken.

In addition to the lotion shops, the health food store was another good source for lotions with nutritional and therapeutic benefits—those known to be good for the skin (e.g., vitamin E, beta-carotene, chamomile, et al). We also had shower gels.

Some other nice scents were the light colognes and body splashes I brought in. The pleasing smells had an added benefit of drawing people to her wheelchair to comment on the nice fragrance. As the years passed, Mother may not have understood what the people were saying, but she enjoyed the company and welcomed them with a smile.

I should add here that the fragrances were not put on to mask any bad smells, for Mother didn't really have any. Even her breath had very little smell. She had led the cleanest of lives; had the sweetest of dispositions; and her colon stayed very regular; so there was nothing malodorous to come out of her skin or mouth, other than some routine garment change. I was amazed. Also, I was surprised at how soft her skin was. It was like a baby's.

Once I read of an Indian Yogi who died in the U.S. A mortician certified that his body didn't begin to decompose for fifty-two days after death. If that actually happened, I imagine the delay was due to his purity. As Bernice's passing closed in, I couldn't help but think that her decomposition would take longer than normal as well.

Cards and Balloons

On holidays, birthdays, and other special occasions, we liked to bring cards and balloons in. We'd read the cards to her and then leave them on her chest of drawers. The helium balloons were colorful, and I usually tied them to the back of her wheelchair. She couldn't see them from her position, but again they would draw other people to her, to comment on the balloons and give her a little more attention. Other times we would tie the balloons to something in her room so that she could always see them.

TV, Nature, Lawrence Welk, and Cole Porter

For comfort and entertainment in the room, we tried a number of things. First, but not foremost, we brought in a TV with VCR. Mother could not operate it at all, so an aide or I would set something up. During the week, I usually put on mild nature programs on commercial-free stations and would leave those on when I left. On Saturday nights, Lawrence Welk was on, and I knew she enjoyed that big band music.

Strangely enough, there were times when I came to visit, and rap videos were playing. She would be lying down usually and not watching. I knew that an aide had been in the room to change her or put her to bed. The music and videos didn't seem to touch her, but the image of her generation and those rap videos coming together was funny—such is America.

Speaking of TVs in a nursing home, I'm reminded of a funny scene in the TV room of a facility I had visited. The TV was one of those giant screens. The residents were at lunch, and someone had then put on a program with a televangelist in Mexico. The preacher was speaking Spanish about twice as fast as I have ever heard it; and, he was at least twice as dramatic as any U.S. televangelist I had seen. He was rolling on the stage and on his knees pleading for this or that. Anyway, I was waiting in the TV area as the aides started bringing in patients from the lunch room. After a few minutes I looked at the faces of the residents, and their expressions were priceless. They seemed to be asking, "Where am I?" "Who is that?" "What's going on?" It's hard enough for dementia patients to grasp what's going on when their native language is used; switch to a foreign language and a flamboyant televangelist, and they really think they're in outer space.

For videos, I brought in tapes that I felt she could relate to, and that would promote a peaceful atmosphere. There were two Lawrence Welk tapes—one was a tribute to the big bands, and the second was a salute to Cole Porter. Then I got a couple of nature tapes—one was a survey and showing of wild birds in their natural habitats, and the second was a beautiful film on butterflies and how to lure them to your backyard.

Butterflies

Butterflies were a theme that I used in other ways as well. On a return trip from Florida, my wife and I stopped at Callaway Gardens in Georgia and visited their butterfly house. It was spectacular with a wondrous variety of butterflies flying all around us in a butterfly-friendly environment. The interior had trees, bushes, and ponds; and the walls were clear glass that let in the sun.

Those butterflies flew happily around us, and it was as though they had invited us to be a part of their world. As I watched the rainbow of thousands of colored wings swirl around us, I thought, "This is what I imagine for Mother. The Alzheimer's disease is just a stifling cocoon from which she will eventually emerge to freedom. She will gain her much-deserved wings and raise joy to a new height."

Before leaving Callaway, we bought a large poster of many different butterflies settling on, and flying around, a pink azalea bush. Later we put this on a wall in her room, so she could always see it—envisioning the beauty and joy of these happy pilots.

Also, I purchased an oversized monarch butterfly made of rubber and painted in perfect detail. I tied this to the back of her wheelchair, so it appeared from the front as though the butterfly was riding on her shoulder. From that position, she couldn't really see it; but other people did and stopped by her wheelchair to say something nice about it. Again, that served a good purpose in having more people stop to talk with her and share a touch and a smile. From a distance, it was always fun to see her wheelchair coming toward me with her trusty friend monarch on her shoulder. If real butterflies had been allowed in the nursing home, I'm sure they would have settled on her shoulder, feeling safe there and realizing that she was as gentle as they were.

Music and Other Soothing Sounds

To provide a calming atmosphere and try to replace the nervous agitation that often accompanies Alzheimer's disease, I tried a few different approaches. First, there were the nature programs on TV and also the white noise from the HEPA air filter. Further, I purchased an electronic simulator of nature sounds: light and heavy rain; storms; the ocean with various levels of waves breaking; and waterfalls. It was effective as long as she didn't get distracted. I took that device home at night because I believe it would have quickly disappeared otherwise.

The Sugar Plum Fairy

For her first Christmas at the nursing home, I wanted to give Mother some symbols that represented the season. There were already decorations in the nursing home itself. The activities department had trees on each floor and boughs or wreaths along the walls.

On Bernice's chest of drawers, I put a miniature Christmas tree which had been a present from my oldest sister some years before. It was a ceramic copy of a full evergreen—about twelve inches high and dotted with little, colored, crystal lights which were inset. The tree carried memories of home, though I'm not sure Mother could recollect who gave it to her, or if it was hers at all. Still, it was pretty, and she appreciated its presence.

Then, I bought another seasonal reminder. It was a small globe on a stand—one of those filled with water and snow flakes on the bottom. When turned upside down, the effect would simulate a nice snowfall. In the center of the globe was a young ballerina on a rotating stand. Beneath the globe in a molded stand was a music box which could be wound up. It played "The Dance of the Sugar Plum Fairy" as the little ballerina did her pirouette while the stand rotated and the snow fell. Mother enjoyed this as I could tell by her smile. It may have brought back memories of long ago, but she didn't say anything. She didn't wind it up herself, as that process was beyond her then. However, she did enjoy listening to the music and watching the young ballerina.

Bedside Brahms

With AD patients, their restlessness makes it more difficult to keep an eye on them and ensure their safety. They often feel out of place in their surroundings and have the need to find their way home—wherever or whatever "home" may be.

In Mother's case, the restlessness included trying to get out of her bed at the nursing home in order to find her way home. Most often this happened at night when no one else was in the room. The worst fear for caregivers in such a situation is that the care recipient will fall and injure themselves; although they may still be technically ambulatory, residents can have a hard time negotiating the process of getting out of bed. The first step to hinder this process is putting side rails on the bed. This will stop some people but not the determined. Bernice tried to climb over the side rails and was discovered by an aide before she made the drop to the floor. Sometimes the aides would remember to put up the side rails, and sometimes they wouldn't; that was another thing I had to keep an eye on.

My thought was to get something which would soothe her restlessness and help her fall asleep. I bought a mobile which was secured to the side rails. It had several arms with various little stuffed animals hanging from them. The arm span was about two feet, and they were about a foot and a half above her face as she lay in bed. This new addition had an added safety benefit. Because of the mobile's position above her, she would get tangled in the arms and hanging animals if she tried to climb over the rails. Just the tangle of things was enough to discourage her at that point. Above the arms were a windup music box and a gear to rotate the arms in a circle. The music box played Brahms's Lullaby. It was really a beautiful thing and just what you might imagine would please a child, especially at bedtime.

When I finished my visit at night, I would tuck the covers up to Bernice's neck, give her a kiss on the forehead and watch her smile. Then I would wind up the music box, and we would start listening to Brahms. In my head I would recall the old words—those she had lightly sung to me long ago—"Rock-a-bye, Rock-a-bye, Rock-a-bye little baby...."

Birdfeeders

Another pleasant distraction I decided to add for Mother were birdfeeders—one for finches and another larger one for other birds. Since she lived on the second floor, supporting arms were needed from mounts on the building; the maintenance men were most helpful in putting those up for us. I believe Bernice got some joy from those additions when the birds stopped by, and she looked from her bed through the windows to the feeders. Looking at them myself, I sometimes thought back to the scene several years earlier when she and I sat on the back porch making bird whistles and laughing.

Post-Caregiving Poem

Last year, almost two years after Mother passed away; I passed by the nursing home one notable night and later wrote the following poem:

Rides in the Night

I passed the old nursing home tonight.
A fire station ambulance was there.
"Who were they for?" I wondered.
"Who would be wheeled out on a stretcher?"

So many years I drove *TO* the nursing home.
Now I drive *BY* the nursing home.
So many times the flashing lights greeted my arrival,
And I would wonder, "Who is it?"
"What's happened to them?"
I would pray, "Let it not be Mother."
"She's suffered enough already."

Sometimes it was for Mother—
Not the flashing lights or sirens,
But a quiet ambulance ride to the hospital,
And the entrance to ER medicine.

I would follow the riders,
Meeting them at the Emergency Room.
Then we began the four-hour wait
That filled numerous nights.

Staying by her side
In an inner room—
A circle of pods,
Each awaiting the doctor's entrance.
Sometimes we just started laughing.

She was brave and without complaints—
No more thought of a cut being stitched
Than yesterday's menu.
High temps., infections, flus, cuts,
Cold bugs circulating like wildfire,
"Change of mental status" or coma—
Or death—
All can summon the carriage to the nursing home.

We wait yet again,
Diverted to another ER this time—
A different hospital
But the same four-hour wait.
Bernice dozes off and on.
I hold her hand to comfort—
A small reassurance to say,
"I'm here, Mother. You're not alone."
The added value of touch
When the mind can't fathom speech.
Maybe a hospital admission,
Maybe a return to the nursing home—
Another night done,
Now a bit of rest before the day's work ahead.

I glance up again and note the ambulance.
Yes, now I'm driving BY the nursing home, not TO it.
I have to remind myself of that.
Our long struggles are over.
We won.
Yet I miss that wonderful person.
Drives often take me by that nursing home.
Sometimes I'm taken back to those years,
Sometimes not.
But a waiting, nighttime ambulance there
Will draw my eyes without choice—
For better or worse,
Some elderly soul is about to leave the building.

CHAPTER 10

LOVE AND LAUGHTER

The entire sum of existence is the magic of being needed
by just one person.
    —Vii Putnam

We learn only from those we love.
    —Johann Wolfgang Von Eckermann
      Conversation with Eckermann

Love cures people—both the ones who give it and the
ones who receive it.
    —Dr. Karl Menninger

Laughter is the closest thing to the grace of God.
    —Karl Barth, Swiss Theologian

D URING THE SPAN OF ONE PERSON'S ALZHEIMER'S DISEASE (AD),
the caregiver and care recipient may share a full spectrum of emotions. As individuals, they can also experience a wide range of feelings.

The common vision—or mental flash—of AD is the sight of a very old person staring out into space. That often occurs at life's end. However, from the time a person begins to show signs of dementia and then gets an AD diagnosis, until he or she reaches the stage of silent stare and final days, there can be a great deal of drama.

Prior to this chapter, I wrote about the difficult emotions— some faced by the care recipient, some by the caregiver, some shared together, some shared by and among the whole family, and some by the individual and community. The dynamics can be as dramatic as anything ever imagined.

*****

Now I turn to the most important emotion and its dynamics—the power and strength of love as experienced by and between care recipient and caregiver, at least as experienced by this caregiver and my care recipient—Bernice Buchanan. In a way, everything written before this chapter is simply a prologue to the story, and everything written after it is an epilogue. Love served as a protective umbrella and provided our best shelter from the almost perpetual storm of Alzheimer's disease.

The journey Mother and I made through the labyrinth of AD was fueled by love in many dynamics—one of which was the addition of laughter whenever possible. Bernice was a fun person and was the first to laugh at herself throughout her life. We shared many a smile and much laughter.

When I first approached caregiving, my attitude toward Mother involved many facets—respect for the person she was and for the exemplary life she had lived; dutiful regard for the person who had brought me into the world; gratitude for all she had done for me in life; and love for a great human being and a good friend.

As we evolved through the disease and caregiving process, it was the love in our friendship that sustained us time and again. While I always loved and respected Mother and felt very comfortable in talking with her, it was our friendship which rose to a much higher level during caregiving.

Happiness and Fun

As her memory became worse, she took the situation in stride. She didn't complain nor demonstrate any self-pity. I had assured her that I would be there for her as long as she needed me, and that gave her comfort. We took it a day at a time. Her sense of humor stayed strong. She found an anonymous poem that spoke of her situation and shared the poem with me. It read as follows:

A Little Mixed Up

Just a line to say I'm living

That I'm not among the dead
Though I'm getting more forgetful
And more mixed up in my head.

For sometimes I can't remember
When I stand at the foot of the stairs
If I must go up for something
Or I've just come down from there.

And before the fridge so often
My poor mind is filled with doubt
Have I just put food away?
Or have I come to take it out?

And there are times when it is dark out
With my hairnet on my head
I don't know if I'm retiring
Or just getting out of bed.

So, if it is my turn to write you
And there's no need in getting sore
I may think that I have written
And don't want to be a bore.

So, remember I do love you
And I wish that you were here
And now it is nearly mail time
So I must say "Good-bye, dear."

There I stood beside the mailbox
With face so very red
Instead of mailing your letter
I had opened it instead. (end of poem)

Mother got such a kick out of this poem. It just goes to show how accepting she was of whatever fate brought her way. She was the eternal optimist. Her motto could have been— good news: we'll enjoy it; bad news: we'll work with it.

One summer afternoon we were sitting on the back patio watching the leaves on the big oak rustle in the wind and just enjoying the day. I saw Mother looking off for a second, and I made the whistle of a cardinal. She turned back to the tree and looked up, saying, "Where is that bird?" I replied, "I don't know." Soon I had to smile, and she caught what had happened and smiled herself. "Oh, you did that," she said. Then, as something else caught my attention, I heard an attempted whistle from behind me. I looked back and saw her lips pursed. She smiled and said, "I can do that, too." We laughed a little bit. Then she said, "We're having fun, aren't we?" I sincerely replied, "Yes, Mother, we're having fun."

If we were talking, or attempting to, one of us might break into a smile and the other would join so that we shared a good laugh. Sometimes, she or I would add, "Boy, that's a good one," referring of course to some joke that was not spoken but was somehow understood. This kept the laughter medicine flowing.

Even well into the final stage of Alzheimer's, we still had fun. She didn't know anyone's name, including mine. She didn't know anyone, except for friendly presences. In my case, she always recognized me as someone close to her, but she couldn't always place me. If she looked puzzled, I'd say, "I'm your son, Mother." And she'd reply, "I know."

Bernice was an innocent who had never been corrupted. She had been stress-tested, and she came out of it completely intact. The world could try as it would and still not compromise Mother. Her character and integrity stayed healthy, and she couldn't, or wouldn't, be diverted. Most importantly, she stayed so intact with joy. Simply put, she knew who she was, and accepted herself happily and humbly.

When I met her friends from the apartment complex, the church or her other groups, they always said to her, "You're so lucky to have your son with you now." She would just smile, nod her head, and say, "Yes, I know." She enjoyed that and so did I.

*****

The disease was no reason to diminish my respect for her in any way. It was quite the contrary— by maintaining her smile and the sparkle in her eye after the times of anguish, she proved to me that her character was stronger than the disease. AD physically attacked her brain, but it didn't break her spirit. That was truly notable, especially as I remember the many AD patients I've seen and known whose spirits seemed to be silenced or tortured by the relentless onslaught of the disease.

Bernice's love for humanity was never broken. Well into final stage AD, she would sit in her wheelchair and still try to help those patients who passed by in sorrow. Another sufferer would be crying as he or she was wheeled by, and Mother—with the compassion showing on her face—would literally reach out with comfort. Bernice could only speak odd syllables at that point but that didn't deter her. She was without pause in her devotion to helping others.

I don't believe I could maintain the composure and selflessness she had. I imagine I'd be wringing my hands and calling to God to relieve the pain and confusion of my mental disintegration. One elderly patient I saw at the nursing home cried out constantly, "Holy Mary, Mother of God! Help me!" That went on for what seemed to be a couple of months. And no amount of comfort or reassurance I tried to give would diminish that lady's recitation or the pleading tone.

In the last few years of her life, when people would ask how Mother was doing, I would always say she was fine. What else can you say? They don't really want to hear about Alzheimer's deterioration. The question put to me the most was, "Does your Mother know you?" To that I would honestly and happily answer, "Our smiles know each other." And they did.

Unconditional Love

The year after my return to Indianapolis, I noticed an ad in the newspaper one day announcing an appearance by Ram Dass at the Murat Theater downtown. He was to give a talk and then have a Q&A on the subject of service in addition to his life and experiences in general. I thought it would be interesting to hear him speak so I purchased a ticket.

Ram Dass (aka Richard Alpert) gained national attention in the mid-1960s when he was involved with Timothy Leary in hallucinogenic research at Harvard. That process seemed to be the manna or magic carpet for many American late adolescents en route to flower power.

Considering that I spent that period in the army and half of that time was overseas, I didn't know much about him or the hallucinogenic movement. I wasn't opposed to the flower children or their accoutrements, but they did seem a bit like dilettantes compared to the serious life of their contemporaries in the military.

In any event, I now felt my curiosity sparked about how he might summarize that period of history and his involvement in it; that is, the other side of the coin. His current interest was in service to others, and I could relate to that. So, I figured it was time to amend my '60s education and see what else he had learned.

He spoke to an audience of over 2,000 people. Then the Q&A began. There were questions on the subject of service to others and also on his particular style of meditation. Then he took my question which was, "Considering all of your experiences in life, which would you consider the single most wonderful and life-altering?" He paused for just a second and then said, "That was when I met my guru and experienced unconditional love." He was smiling as he apparently drifted back to that encounter.

*****

I wasn't exactly sure what unconditional love was, and I still imagine that each person must define it for himself or herself. The thoughts or characteristics that come to mind are: unqualified acceptance, true friendship, strong affection.

One experience I did have in the early 1980s had to qualify in that special category. That event was one which William James in his classic *The Varieties of Religious Experience*[1] had defined as a "peak experience" or mystical revelation. Actually, my experience was on Tuesday morning, October 12, 1982. I awoke about 6 AM and felt absolutely perfect. I thought that I must still be asleep and dreaming. I stayed in bed, kept my eyes open and marveled at how wonderful this feeling was. Imagining that it would pass when I got out of bed to get ready for work, I was happily surprised to note the feeling didn't diminish. There was not the slightest bit of anxiety, fear, insecurity, or any thread of negative emotion; nor was it a feeling of jubilance. It was a feeling beyond description, beyond the beyond. I felt that I was part of everybody and everything, and they were part of me. It was acceptance. It was complete understanding. It was bliss.

I worked in a high pressure environment—a type studio providing pre-press layouts for the advertising agencies. Urban ad agencies, exemplified by Madison Avenue, are known far and wide for their pressured environments. But, in fact, they just transferred that pressure to the studio doing their layouts. My temperament could handle that pressure better than most people could, but the pressure could still get to one on some level. It was always in the air.

During my experience, even that pressure couldn't touch me. I was walking and working in a state of grace. An invisible protective barrier surrounded me, and nothing negative could enter nor even be recognized. I was one with everyone and everything. I went about my work with absolute, perfect, loving calm. I thought, "If this state is Heaven—life after death—then I am ready to die...right now...this moment. Take me now, Lord." There simply could not be a more perfect bliss. Its origin and operation could only be based in a universal, indiscriminate love—unconditional love. I have read of others having this peak experience and yet many of them wouldn't even talk about it, or did so only with hesitation for fear of being labeled off-balance or crazy or some such nonsense. I never hesitated to talk about that experience. I believe in sharing good things—most importantly, sharing the knowledge that such wonderful states are possible at all.

The feeling/state did diminish slightly and progressively during the day. When I woke up the next morning, it was gone. At that point, my first thought was gratitude to God that I had been allowed to experience it, and for so long. My second thought was trying to figure how to get it back. I tried to factor in a ton of conditions and circumstances to get it again. Finally, I realized it was not something which could be ordered or arranged. It was just a gift and had to be accepted that way.

Someone asked me if it was like the calm of a high-powered drug, an analgesic or some such thing. No, I replied, it was worlds beyond anything artificial. I had experienced a fair amount of morphine during a severe kidney stone attack, and the light relief of morphine was like absolutely nothing compared to the power of that all-encompassing, natural bliss I had experienced.

So that was my perception and experience of unconditional love. I've known times of great joy and happiness, but the experience of bliss was in another category altogether. As important as having that experience was the complete realization that such states are actually possible. When someone once started preaching to me about the afterlife and going to Heaven, I simply replied, "I've been to Heaven, and it is most wonderful." That stopped the preaching.

Caregiving and Unconditional Love

If most fortunate during the caregiving experience, the caregiver and care recipient will experience and share unconditional love. This can happen in certain instances. This does not preclude the intermittent presence of anxieties, fears, anger, helplessness, and other feelings that are bound to appear in one form or another, at one time or another. However, one taste of unconditional love will overshadow or neutralize all those other sentiments that represent the frailty of the human condition.

For anyone who has tasted the nectar of unconditional love, the lures of common life hold no interest. Gold, jewels, trips around the world, trips into outer space, being desired by the most alluring sex idols, even immortality—all fall by the wayside. In reality, those objects of desire are simply shortcomings in our ability to find peace within ourselves. Unconditional love has no equal. I believe that unconditional love is the touch of God.

Again, what is unconditional love? Your opinion is probably as valid as mine or that of anyone else who has ever tried to define it. For me, another definition may be to love without thought of return or simply to love without conditions; easier said than done. Why? By appearance, love should be simple—just allow it to happen. Actually, everything that bonds us to people as individuals and to groups with restricted membership is something which stands in the way of unconditional love—at least universal unconditional love.

When we set aside our needs—the need to belong, the need to survive, the need to be loved—then we're on the path to real love. When we take that leap of faith to identify with all living things, we begin to understand the bond that connects us all. When we stop thinking me first, then we're taking a step in the right direction.

However, for now let's stick to the application at hand—the caregiving of one person for another who is not able to take care of himself or herself; more specifically, how to feel and hold this love when you are being severely taxed by the disease which is overtaking your loved one.

I find that real love comes with practice. You start with a general feeling of devotion toward a person. This may be based on your feeling that it is the right thing to do or it may be in reaction to the things this person has done for you. That is a start. Then, in caregiving, you begin to face the hurdles. Your strength of purpose is tested constantly—perhaps by the disease as it affects your loved one, or by lack of support and antagonism from other family members, or by the lack of help from society, or by the struggle to maintain the basic needs of your own existence. All of this may be facing you while you carry out your caregiving, your personal commitment, your chosen obligation, this act of love.

*****

In my case, or I should say our case since the feeling was interactive between caregiver and loved one, joy was closely associated with the good love I felt. I couldn't speak for Mother's feelings, as it was harder—no, impossible—to get any understandable verbal response; however, her facial responses said so much more than the spoken word.

When I saw the sparkle in her eye, when I saw her smile, when I saw the childlike look of wonder on her face, it was a great boost for me. That signified her spirit being fully intact and present. The syllables coming out of her mouth made no sense, but that was irrelevant.

A few years ago, a strange thing happened as she mentally drifted farther away. At some point I began calling her Mama. All my life I had called her Mother, without variation. That seemed casual, friendly, and respectful. I'm not sure where that new change of address came from.

The only previous reference made to "Mama" was made by her in 1994. Losing touch with time and place, she asked me, "Where's Mama?" I hesitated but then carefully told her, "Your mother passed away a long time ago. She's buried in Illinois." At this, Bernice started crying, in pain, and said, "Oh, no! Oh, no!" It was heartbreaking for me. Her mother had passed away over 40 years earlier. That scene happened a couple of times before I realized that I had to say something different. I wouldn't lie to her, but I had to avoid that harsh reality again and again. Next time, when she asked me, "Where's Mama?" I simply replied, "She's in Illinois." Mother then had a hurt look on her face, but she didn't cry. Eventually she stopped asking.

Then we had to go through the same experience with Papa; again, the heartbreaking loss, again my modification. Then she would ask for her brother Bernard. He was alive and living in Florida, so I just mentioned that he was living in Florida. She seemed to feel the distance but no tears. Still, she would ask for Bernard time and again. Her brother Bernard was about a year and a half older than Bernice. Strangely enough, he had developed Alzheimer's at about the same time as Mother. Also, when I spoke at that time with Aunt Evelyn, Bernard's wife and caregiver, I found out that he had been asking for Bernice, just as she had called out for him.

During those most stressful moments—a stage of the disease which comes and then passes away—a person often calls out for a loved one from the past, an anchor or protector, perhaps from childhood. Bernice was very much in need of love, comfort, and assurance when she asked for her parents and brother at those times. She was in the middle stage of AD and having a hard episode of inner chaos and anguish. She was reverting back to her childhood security figures.

Love Among The Lepers

Thirty-six years ago I experienced a good example, and most exceptional atmosphere, of love. It was like a pervasive cloud that covered and then converted you.

While a soldier and stationed in northeastern Thailand, I made a trip with a couple of buddies to the little mountain city of Chieng Mai in northwestern Thailand. During our three days in Chieng Mai, some missionaries took us well out into the countryside and mountain jungle to experience a lot more. First we went to a little artisan village where the people made ornate silver cups and other pieces, as well as beautifully decorated bamboo umbrellas. Next we went to visit a hill tribe and spoke with the villagers through an interpreter about their lives.

Finally, we went to call on a leper colony. Though approaching the village with some apprehension, I went away feeling wonderful. As I imagine in all countries, lepers in Thailand faced a rough life. They would have to leave their home village and somehow fend for themselves. They were social pariahs. In addition to the immediate decay of their bodies, they had the subsequent burden of feeling banished, abandoned, and worthless, I imagine.

Not so in the leper colony. In that colony, they were accepted, encouraged and loved. They made friends. They found mates. They learned skills. They received medical care to treat their wounds and had infected limbs removed as necessary. They beamed with the love and respect that flourished in that village. Some of their skills were as artisans, and they sold their work to visitors and to merchants in Chieng Mai.

The missionaries told us of American medical personnel who donated some time working in the colony. One volunteer was a doctor—a surgeon, I believe—who donated two weeks to the colony. Then he began to donate two weeks a year; then six weeks a year; then six months a year; and finally he moved there to serve full-time.

I imagine that doctor was dedicated to service in the manner of Dr. Schweitzer. He may simply have recognized the higher calling. The sense of purpose and satisfaction and profound gratitude from the patients would have been pretty strong lures. However, perhaps the crowning point in his decision was the atmosphere of love in that remote colony. As is often said, "God is Love." And what better life could be led than to be following your sense of purpose, be appreciated, and also surrounded by love.

Love at the Nursing Home

Before entering specific instances of love that Mother and I shared at the nursing home, I want to mention another example that I witnessed. That event was truly notable.

It was Christmastime, and that is generally a joyful period in all settings. At the nursing home, there were always more visitors—family and outside groups (e.g., Boy Scouts, Girl Scouts, Sunday school classes, singing groups, etc.).

The night was cold with blowing snow as I approached the front door of the facility and looked through the door window into the front reception room. There were about fifty people of all ages, and everyone was happy and hugging each other. I've seldom seen such powerful unity in so many people. I couldn't hear anything at all because there were two solid entrance doors, and any sound would be blocked. The first door opened into a porch for shaking off the weather before entering the facility itself.

Entering the inner porch, I still didn't hear anything as I looked through the glass door and to the very happy gathering. Assuming that they were speaking little and low among the hugs, I opened the second door and entered the front room where the group was about fifteen feet away.

There was absolute, total silence in the room—not that they stopped talking on my entrance for they didn't turn nor acknowledge me in any way. Immediately, I recognized that it was part of NH #3's deaf population in addition to other deaf people—including Boy Scouts—from the outside world.

It struck me that they were all so happy. Many kids—including adolescents—are uncomfortable in a nursing home. Something in their faces will usually signal it. Not so in this case—they were a unified, joyous, loving group of people.

Perhaps their joyful love was in the bonding of the common challenge they shared. Perhaps for the young ones, it was seeing role models who made it through their lives with the hardship they themselves had. Perhaps for the old ones, it was seeing the young people who cared about them. In any event, it was truly a scene of fluid love that included everyone there.

There must be many people like myself who are spiritually uplifted just by witnessing such an event or exchange. Just by being in the environment, one feels wrapped up in the happiness and love of the gathering.

Joy between Friends

More than individual instances, Mother and I shared a steady flow of love at the nursing home. I don't remember our having a down side. The disease was more advanced, and the blessing of that was that Bernice's anguish diminished a great deal. There were a few scenarios that consistently lit up our lives. This is not to say that the nursing home is generally a joyous environment, but there are standout moments.

This scenario started when I stepped out of the elevator and saw my mother. She was about twenty feet away in her wheelchair and sitting by the nurses' station. She may have been looking at someone in the chair next to her and trying to communicate, or she could have been looking a bit downcast as she tried to put it all together—herself, her environment, how she got there, where would she go from there. It is difficult to say how much of that is being pondered by an AD patient, since we don't know what faculties are left within the brain. Suffice it to say that the downward-cast look carried a bit of sadness but no self-pity.

I waited by the elevator and faced her, waiting for Bernice to look up and see me. When she did, a smile spread across her face—a smile that was more valuable than a truckload of gold and gems. It was not just *a* smile, or even *her* smile, as her smile always showed some joy. Much beyond, her smile at that time was a mix of happiness, love, gratitude, and peace.

As I walked toward her, I saw her world brighten a great deal. And when her world brightened, the whole room could be affected positively. It was probably the combination of smile and sparkle in her eyes and the evident love she had for people as a whole. The staff and other residents who witnessed that took note of her reaction as I came in. Usually one nurse or aide would say, "Look how happy she is!" or something else to that effect. It's notable when a resident beams with happiness.

For my part, the reward was like feeling on top of the world. Her look seemed to regard me as a savior, liberator, and a soul who truly cared about her — cared more about her than anyone else did. I believe she saw me as a tall beacon of light and love in an atmosphere that must have yielded much confusion and frustration amidst the lighter moments of hands-on caring and group activities. At least that's what her smile said to me.

The joy she projected then was amazing. It was as though I was liberating her from a detention center, or adopting and reclaiming her from an orphanage for the elderly unwanted. I saw the happiness a puppy must feel when someone picks it up at the pound to give it a loving home. Somewhere in her heart and soul the message was constructed to facially demonstrate, "I'm cared about and loved and wanted, and someone is going to save me from this oblivion of wandering, sad souls." That was how it came across.

Of course I couldn't really save her at that point, at least not in the respect of taking her home and caring for her there. Her needs then were far beyond my capabilities. The best I could do was to give her a temporary reprieve during our daily visits. The only complete saving she would experience was when she was finally liberated and passed into the next life. In this existence, her brief, special flights of joy ended when I entered the elevator and the doors closed behind me. Not long after the elevator went down, she must have returned to wondering where she was and who these people were. The staff told me she could be cheerful and spiritually helpful to her fellow residents at many other times, but that her joy was never the same as when I arrived.

In terms of benefit, I enjoyed the visits at least as much as she did. We enjoyed each other's company and were good friends. Perhaps most importantly, we both liked to laugh—sometimes it was more of a giggle or a light chuckle, but the smiles on our faces and sparkle in our eyes spoke of a common understanding. The understanding itself was probably the realization that the gift of laughter was good medicine in overcoming the harder parts of life.

Until a couple of years before, she would interrupt her laughter to say the classic line, "That's a good one!" When I realized she was no longer able to make those words or put that phrase together, I started saying it for her. After we laughed for a little while, I would smile and say, "That's a good one!" I continue to do that now—part of my inheritance, I guess.

*****

I remember another scene as I got off the elevator one evening. This time was close to the end of her life. Dinner was over, and Mother was sitting in her wheelchair against the wall with a lady on each side of her in their wheelchairs. To the left, Ester was muttering something to herself with her head staring at her lap and her eyes closed. On the right, Evelyn's eyes were closed, and she was quiet. Mother had part of her smile and was looking to share it with one of her neighbors. They didn't even know she was there. Three eighty-something women whose systems were closing down for the night, as the dark winter black was complete outside.

From the elevator to her wheelchair was about twenty feet. I whispered softly, "Mother." No response. Then a little louder, "Mother." She looked up. Her lips mouthed the word, "Mother." Then she said it aloud, "Mother." She looked to the left, saw me, and a big smile came to her face—a smile cherished by so many friends and family, loved for its honest sincerity and aliveness with the sparkling eyes, like a child at Christmastime.

The smile was nearly toothless now, and it was more precious than ever. She was beyond any inhibitions about missing teeth. She was beyond knowing what teeth were. She was almost beyond making any words, though they would come out occasionally. Now it was mostly syllables. The slightly puzzled look couldn't quite connect them to anything. She wasn't frustrated about it, just a little curious for a moment.

She looked at me again, and her smile broadened. She knew who I was. At least she knew that I was someone who loved her and was here for her. I was her closest human connection since we had spent the last ten years together tightly bonded. I don't think she knew my name, nor did she likely know that I was her son; that's hard to be sure of in analyzing the Alzheimer's brain. However, she knew that I was very caring of her. She also felt that she was safe with me. I was thankful for that much by that point.

I hugged her and gave her a kiss on the cheek. Another smile from her. "Mother, let's go get a piece of chocolate." That didn't register with her then, though the "c" word usually brought a smile and a "Yes!"

Wheeling her to her room, I noticed the aides taking other residents to their rooms to put them to bed. Inside Bernice's room, I got the chocolate and fed it to her in little pieces. Her mouth opened for them like a little bird receiving bits from the Mother. And this was the case now—I was the Mother and she the child. It had been this way for awhile with her instincts becoming increasingly primal. In that vein, I think about the times I put a flower to her nose to smell, but she would reach for it with open mouth. Food or sustenance must be our most basic calling, and she had regressed to that response.

To my happiness, she still retained so much of the joy she had shown throughout her life. The photo printed in chapter three of Bernice at her four-year-old birthday party shows it all. She was surrounded by her friends, waving a little American flag and buoyant with that childlike happiness. God helped her to keep that joy throughout her life—a life that was not without its trials and tribulations. Still, she always had that inner reservoir to fall back on.

Her head started to nod then. I hugged her again, told her how much I loved her, said goodnight, and left the room. Outside, I told the aide that it was bedtime for Bernice.

Children and Pets

Some visitors that were always welcome and most always brought joy to nursing home residents were children and pets. I would often recommend to the activities director to bring in as many children's groups as possible. The holiday period of Thanksgiving to New Year's Day was when most kids visited. They had Cub Scouts, brownies, Girl Scouts, Boy Scouts, Sunday school classes, elementary school classes, etc. They would come in to mix with the residents, or do a group singing, or deliver holiday cards to each resident.

The smallest children seemed to be the most welcome by the residents. I'm not sure what the primary appeal to the residents was. Perhaps in kids the residents reflected on themselves at that time in life, a happier time with full strength and a full life ahead. They may have also been lured to a remembered time of innocence in life.

For Bernice, the contact with children and pets, especially children, was another chance to share love. When Mother saw young children, an extra sparkle would come to her eye with an additional smile and chuckle as well. I never saw any adult who could nourish the spirit of a child more wonderfully than my mother. She related to them in a most special way. This had always been the case, and it didn't change or diminish when she got Alzheimer's.

A Special Little Girl

While children were appreciated by the residents at the nursing home, the kids were often uncomfortable in being there. I assume the sight of so many old and disabled people, mostly in wheelchairs, was scary to the kids. They probably wanted to say hello and then get out of there. I could see kids trying to hold their smiles, but I also noticed many smiles soon beginning to crack in response to some unknown anxiety. The elderly are not treated well in America—especially the elderly disabled who are hidden away—so it was not surprising to see kids in the nursing home looking a bit fearful.

One night I saw a pretty little girl get off the elevator with her mother. The girl was about seven and the Mother no more than thirty. They had come to visit the little girl's grandfather. This girl was not afraid of the old people. She was actually drawn to them. On her own, she began going around saying hello to the residents in their wheelchairs before the mother took her in to see the grandfather.

When the mother and child came out into the general area again, the little girl came over to where Bernice and I were. The girl's mother was at the nurse's station speaking with a nurse. Bernice's gaze was drawn to the little girl like a magnet, as was the little girl to Bernice. She and the girl, both with smiles and dancing eyes, looked deep into each other's eyes and didn't say a word. That seemed to last almost a full minute. It was strange and beautiful. There seemed to be a special understanding between the 87-year-old lady with dementia and the 7-year-old, simple girl. I thought of the Hindu practice of the guru passing shakti or power to the disciple. In this case, it appeared as one loving spirit soon to leave this life that passed on something to another loving spirit who had recently entered this life. Regardless of the extreme age difference, Bernice and the little girl were similar souls. It appeared that despite Mother's dementia and the little girl's simplicity, the two souls met and communicated on a higher plane. It was really something for me to experience.

The next night I spoke with the girl's mother. She told me that the little girl really did love old people. Sometimes it was hard to drag her away when it was time to go home. Since I was always looking for ways to make Bernice's existence there more pleasant, I told the mother I had an uncommon proposal. I would pay her daughter $10 an hour to spend time with Bernice, all according to the girl's schedule, no matter how much or how little time spent. The mother thought about it, then thanked me but said that her daughter couldn't spend much time there since she needed to get to bed early for school. She was a precious little girl, and she and Bernice would have had many good times together.

*****

Sometimes I couldn't get to the nursing home until Mother was already in bed. I would go in to find her still awake, and then sit and talk with her, or to her. I would make sure the blankets were tucked up to her neck. I felt like a parent tucking in their child at night. Then I would make sure Kermit the Frog was lying next to her with his head on the pillow and looking up at the ceiling with Mother. Occasionally, I would touch one of her toes through the blanket and say, "This little piggy went to the market, and this little piggy..." She would get a big chuckle out of that. Another time when leaving, I would smile and say, "Sleep tight, and don't let the bedbugs bite." Then she'd smile and say, almost seriously, "Oh, you…"

I Love You

Women realize something early in life that men are simply slower to grasp—the concept and value of love and the declaration of love. This is not principally a gender difference resulting from hormones, but more the result of training and role expectations.

Perhaps the closest balance of sincerity between man and woman in using the term "I love you" would be on their wedding day or honeymoon. The world is awaiting them, and everything is so optimistic and promising. There are no threats of survival in the air, nothing to diminish their joy. Beyond marriage or partnership bonding, there are at least equal, if not better, opportunities to express our love—whether vocally or by other action.

Think of the different forms of love we are exposed to in our lifetime—parental love, maternal love, paternal love, brotherly love, sisterly love, filial love, humanitarian love, romantic love, self love, and on. While those listed types of love include human-to-human relationships, there are of course other loving interactions. There is the love for our pets which is often stronger than the love we have for other people. Then we may have a love for other animals, perhaps all the animals in the world. There is the love for plants and trees—those that nourish our bodies, and those that nourish our souls. There is a love of the earth—the GAIA principle (seeing the earth as a conscious entity). There is also a love of life. And finally, there is a love of love.

Far more important than defining the type of love is the ability to understand the quality and significance of love. When we hear the term, "God is Love," we notice that there is no qualifier added (e.g., "God is Paternal Love" or "God is Brotherly Love").

We may start as babies or children with the seed of maternal love. With that assurance from our mother that we are lovable, we can begin to build confidence and strength and a realization that love is an attitude which makes us feel good. Hopefully, that seed sprouts and grows and flourishes. Then we are able to extend the love we receive toward others with whom we come in contact or toward humanity as a whole. At least that would be the ideal.

If we lived in a secure and worry-free environment all our lives, we could work more pointedly toward nourishing and sharing our love, making it a principal focus as we make our way through life. However, society doesn't recognize love as a viable primary goal, so we put it on the back burner, relegate it to a darker and colder spot when we take on the more aggressive enterprises like war and other loveless businesses.

*****

Caregiving provided an opportunity to act completely out of love for another person. This love was expressed in various ways and evolved to what I consider one of the highest forms—the joyful giving and receiving between two friends who are devotedly committed to each other's welfare and the well-being of humanity as a whole. It was a chance to give back in kind to one who had given me so much, perhaps more than anyone else on earth. An important example of this demonstration of love was in saying, "I love you." Our family didn't use that phrase very much. We loved each other, most often acted in loving ways, and seldom felt antagonism against each other. We felt a lot of joy together and had strong emotions. However, we just didn't often use the phrase "I love you." That was a general description of our family behavior. In reality, "I love you" is just a term—just three words. It indicates affection and sincerity, but the degree of those qualities is best interpreted by watching the countenance of the speaker, listening to his or her heart.

As the AD began to increasingly develop in Mother, I found myself starting to say "I love you." I believe this started naturally as a way to assure her that I was there for her and always would be. This increased her sense of security and being grounded while the Alzheimer's was destroying the pathways of logic in her brain.

When Mother went to the nursing home, I increased the love confirmations. At least twice a day I would tell her I loved her. Sometimes she would be shy and silent, but the declaration would bring a smile to her face. Mostly, she sincerely replied to me, "I love you, too." As the disease attacked her verbal abilities, words dropped from her reply. Over time, "I love you, too" changed to "Love you, too" then to "Love you" then to "Love" and finally to "Uv" when she could speak no longer. After that, she replied with a happy smile and finally a beatific smile.

*****

My mother loved to laugh. It was always laughing with people but never at anyone. An exception would be laughing at herself; or laughing with a friend who was laughing at himself or herself; or laughing at a professional comedian who tickled her funny bone—for example, Red Skelton. She would never laugh where it might hurt someone; nor, do I think, would Red Skelton. Interestingly enough, he was also a Hoosier. Mother and he were born in the same year, but she outlived him by five years.

She always stayed with her core moral values about life while still being able to laugh at herself and not let any hard times control her. Her principal advice might be, "Just do your best." I never saw any evidence of self-pity on her part. Her modus operandi was simply maintaining her faith and trying to do the right thing.

Love, laughter, and smiles were the priceless gifts that aided us through the relentless progression of Alzheimer's disease. When so many other poor souls fell by the wayside, we had respites filled with love and laughter. They were the fuel to help our spirits soar whenever possible.

CHAPTER 11

A TIME TO DIE

For what is it to die, but to stand in the sun and melt into the wind? And when the Earth has claimed our limbs, then we shall truly dance.
   —Kahlil Gibran

Death is not extinguishing the light; it is putting out the lamp because dawn has come.
   —Rabindranath Tagore

Be of good cheer about death and know this as a truth— that no evil can happen to a good person, either in life or after death.
   —Socrates

ON JULY 31, 2001, MOTHER WAS SENT TO THE HOSPITAL DUE TO her "change in mental status." She was checked in around 1 PM, and I was notified at work. I went to the hospital and found her still unconscious at 3 PM with an IV in her arm. Dehydration and infection had taken a toll.

Change in mental status in this case meant lethargic to the point of letting her head drop into her lap...as though asleep and unable to wake. I had seen this condition a number of times, and I assumed that it was the result of a urinary tract infection (UTI). (Lab results confirmed this.)

When the nurse came in to check on her, I introduced myself and gave her a note with my phone number. She noticed that I had

Mother listed as "no code" (do not resuscitate) and asked if I had further instructions concerning nutrition and hydration. "No," I replied, "Mother and I only talked about the use of respirators and other mechanical aids to prolong life. We didn't cover nutrition and hydration."

Then she left, and I continued watching Mother. After two hours, she awoke, looked around, and smiled at me. The IV glucose had done its job, and she was rehydrating. We had another hour together before I left.

On the way out, I spoke with her nurse, asking for more information on what she'd said about withholding nutrition and hydration as related to the dying process. She said that by keeping the person comfortable, a dying patient would not suffer at all from lack of food and water. By visual and machine monitoring, a nurse could detect any discomfort or stresses and take appropriate measures to relieve them...with involvement from a doctor as needed.

This nurse and others on the unit had been oriented in-house recently by a hospice admitting nurse. She was impressed with the orientation and suggested that I speak with the hospice nurse to learn more.

At that point, I mentioned to her an end-of-life, food-and-water case I was familiar with. It went as follows—

I knew a retired RN whom I'll call Susan. She also had a Mother with end-stage Alzheimer's disease (AD) who had ended up in the hospital with an infection and was in and out of consciousness. The antibiotics weren't working, and she was in the active dying process with perhaps a week to live. As her mother's guardian, and having consulted with hospice, Susan chose at that point for her mother's care to eliminate nutrition, and just stick with palliative measures.

Her mother's hospital doctor strongly disagreed with her on this, as he wanted to continue nutrition and hydration—food and water. The former nurse still said no, and stuck to orders for palliative treatment. Every day for her mother's remaining week of life, the doctor and/or a unit nurse would persistently ask Susan if she had changed her mind and now wanted to have her mother fed. Every day she replied no.

Susan's mother died quite peacefully following a week in which the final body stresses had been eliminated by the palliative treatment. A couple days after the death, Susan went back to the hospital to pick up her mother's things. As she spoke with someone at the nurse's station,

Susan saw the head nurse off to the side; she was speaking in a low voice to a new nurse on the ward, saying, "That's the woman who let her mother starve to death."

According to Susan, that whole episode took place at a major hospital in Indianapolis in the mid-1990s. I was surprised to hear Susan's account of the doctor's persistent attempts to change the end-of-life choices the daughter had made. She was her mother's guardian and had been entrusted with the power to make these important medical decisions for her mother—period. These are difficult, painful decisions to begin with; to have the attending doctor and a nurse try to change her orders every day made Susan's role even more difficult. Susan was a calm and dispassionate narrator with a clear account..

I believe most doctors and nurses would not act that way—that is, the case of what Susan experienced. I believe that the vast majority of doctors would honor the medical decisions of the patient or guardian without repeatedly trying to impose their own medical choices on the guardian. In Indiana, the law requires that. However, without official paperwork, end-of-life decisions can be contestable. Further, if a patient ends up in a controlling hospital, the staff doctor may still try to impose his or her agenda on the guardian and/or patient, even after other health care decisions have been made.

After I finished relaying that whole past episode to my mother's nurse, she was stunned by Susan's reported experience.

*****

The major lesson to be learned from Susan's experience is this—above all, everyone should have an Advance Directive form filled out with your wishes for medical treatment in the event you can no longer make medical decisions for yourself. Speak with your doctor about this. I filled out a Living Will form as well. Indiana state law gives us a choice of three forms: 1) Health Care Representative (HCR) designation; 2) Living Will; or 3) Life-Prolonging Procedures Declaration. The HCR form designates someone to make medical decisions for you in the event you may not be able to do so for yourself. The Living Will form declares your preferred medical treatment if you are unable to communicate, and you have an incurable condition, death is expected soon, or the use of life-prolonging procedures would serve only to prolong dying. The Life-Prolonging Procedures Declaration is a declaration

that a person wants any treatment available to keep him or her alive under such conditions. The blank forms should be available at your doctor's office. They should also be available at hospitals. There is no need
for a lawyer to complete them. They do have to be notarized, and that
was done at my doctor's office. A copy of your chosen form(s) should
be kept in your medical records. The original forms should be kept by
you with another copy for your HCR. Without an official document, the
matter can become far more complicated and could end up in court with
family members fighting for guardianship. That is the reality.

Hospice

The nurse gave me the hospice phone number, and I called the
hospice nurse to set up an appointment. She was very accommodating—as were all hospice personnel—and agreed to meet me at Mother's
nursing home. My hope was to get Mother signed up and have her benefit by the extra care hospice provides.

Prior to my personal experience with hospice, I thought of it
only as providing pain relief to people with a terminal illness. No one in
my immediate family had used their services, so I had no previous exposure. When I thought of hospice, I imagined people at a dedicated live-
in facility where everyone was close to death, or patients who chose to
die at home and used hospice services there.

During Mother's stay at NH #3, there were a few residents who
used hospice services. Hospice personnel visited them at the facility.
From one of their family members, I learned that a person must be diagnosed with six months or less to live in order to qualify for hospice
services. Further, the services went beyond pain control to include
additional care—from personal touch and conversation to manicures
and anything that would make the patient's remaining time more
comfortable.

On first hearing of the hospice services years earlier, I had
hoped to get Mother enrolled. Unfortunately, it can be difficult to get a
six-months-or-less diagnosis for advanced dementia patients—even end-
stage Alzheimer's sufferers. Stages of AD do not accurately indicate
remaining lifespan. I've read that lifespan remaining after initial AD
diagnosis can range from two to twenty years. Her doctor now couldn't
make the required six-month terminal diagnosis during our first applica-

tion for hospice, so I dismissed the idea and concentrated instead on the day-to-day matters of her care and comfort. Time passed.

Now, I was about to meet Stephanie— an RN and hospice admitting nurse. We had arranged to meet at the nursing home when Mother was back from the hospital. We had our discussion, and I felt very comfortable with her. In order for hospice to know as much as possible about Mother and subsequently provide the best services, I told her of Mother's life and then our last ten years together through the Alzheimer's journey. Then, she told me about hospice treatment and the type of services involved.

First of all, hospice provides palliative care, not aggressive, curative care. In fact, if you pursue aggressive, curative care, you cannot be in hospice. They will work with you in terms of the curative concept. If the patient can stay at the facility and take antibiotics as opposed to being taken to the hospital for more extensive treatment, then the patient can stay in hospice.

Palliative—as in palliative care—is defined in the Cambridge Dictionary as, "a drug or medical treatment that reduces pain without curing the cause of the pain."

As applied to Bernice, palliative care would not require real physical pain medication at this point. The only prescription medicine would possibly be a light tranquilizing agent as needed (PRN). The aim—as it should be—was to quell excessive anxiety or anguish without dulling the senses any more than necessary.

A more objective description of Mother's first hospice care plan involved the following. A hospice RN would stop by twice a week to briefly check Bernice's condition and review her chart for any recent nursing notes. A home health aide would be by twice a week to bathe her and check her overall hygiene. If possible, a hospice volunteer would be by to spend some time with her—time that included doing Mother's nails; or taking her outdoors for a wheelchair ride by the lake; or just holding her hand and talking to her. Finally, a chaplain would be available as his schedule permitted.

I asked Stephanie about the nutrition and hydration issues. The withholding of these life essentials—especially water—implies suffering to most people, including me. She assured me that there is no suffering by withholding food and water as the patient's stresses are managed in order to keep them comfortable. To the contrary, providing food—and even water—just prolong the dying process.

Mother was over the infection now and back at the facility. I took Stephanie in to meet her, and we all spent some time together as Stephanie watched the dynamics between Mother and me—the joy we often shared together through smiles that spoke the same language and always had.

Stephanie and I left Bernice's room, and I signed the paperwork allowing her to be examined by their staff. "Part of our job," said Stephanie "is to take some of the load off your shoulders." I was looking forward to that. Hospice could be helpful as an extra set of eyes monitoring Mother's care when I wasn't there.

When we were through, I walked Stephanie back to her car and received one of those treats which make a caregiver's life a little easier. As she started to get in her car, she turned, looked me in the eye and said, "I want to tell you something, but I don't want to embarrass you. I have an eighteen-month-old son. I hope he grows up to be much like you." I was quite flattered, and all I could say was "Thank you." It may seem immodest to mention that; however, the point is to let readers know that some nice words can be most rewarding to the caregiver— they can make the difference in how a caregiver is able to handle the stressful challenges that face them day after day, whether at their own home or in the nursing home.

The next step would be for me to meet with the hospice social worker and the visiting nurse who would examine Mother. Sharon, the social worker, was available as a facilitator if problems should arise with Mother's care. Lastly, the hospice doctor would be notified so she could make her own exam. The doctor's exam was the determining factor of the patient's eligibility for hospice.

*****

All was done. Mother was diagnosed to have less than six months remaining and subsequently accepted into the hospice program. That was a reality signpost for me to face. Even having been through ten years of AD together and knowing that Bernice couldn't have long to go, it's another wakeup call when being told by a doctor that your loved one has less than six months to live.

Bernice's body was simply worn out. Her immune system was faltering and more susceptible to infections—principally UTIs which plagued women patients more often in nursing homes. It was amazing that she had lasted so long.

I told the nurses at NH #3 that Mother was then enrolled in hospice. They agreed with me on the choice of adding hospice care; it helped lighten their load. Although they voiced agreement, each nurse seemed to do it quietly. I was to learn that nursing home administration can be "not so receptive" to having hospice in the facility.

Why would the nursing home administration not want the supplemental care provided by hospice? It seems to be a matter of control—medical and administrative control. When a nursing home patient is enrolled in hospice, hospice is in charge of his or her services. The nursing home becomes a subcontractor. They receive full monthly resident fees per normal, but they then receive them from the hospice organization. More importantly, any additional medical services (e.g., physical, occupational or speech therapy) must be approved by hospice before proceeding. Perhaps it might be best described as an uneasy alliance. Still, everyone appeared to interact professionally, and I don't believe Mother suffered any diminished care from nursing home staff because of it.

End-Stage Care

One medical research report on appropriate health care for end-stage dementia used a survey of professional caregivers and family caregivers.[1] There were five levels of care, from level one of do everything possible to save the demented person's life to level five which was simply palliative—comforting the patient and controlling their pain. Palliative care was seen as preferable to aggressive care by the majority of respondents.

The majority—90% of family members and 91% of professionals—felt hospice care was appropriate in end-stage. On the question of whether hospice should be in an institution or at home, professionals, when told that a family member could be at home to care for the person, felt that home was the better choice. Family members felt that hospice in an institution was the better choice.

End-stage dementia was defined as: 1) Needs complete assistance with eating and toileting; 2) Can't do any of the things which used to make him/her happy; 3) Can no longer recognize you or other loved ones; 4) Cannot talk anymore; and 5) Is suffering from medical complications of dementia such as: falls, urinary incontinence, or pneumonia.

The majority of professionals and family in that study were opposed to tube feeding in end-stage dementia.

I'll return to level one for a moment. The full conditions of level one ("Do everything to prolong life") were "No matter what happens, do everything possible to keep the person alive including: treat any illnesses, such as hypertension and pneumonia, that occur. If the patient can't eat, use tube feeding. When tube feeding is used, a tube for food is put down the nose to the stomach, or directly through the stomach wall. If the patient has a heart attack and the heart stops beating, try to restart the heart including the use of an electrical shock to the chest to try to start the heart beating again. If the patient has difficulty breathing, use a respirator. Respirators are machines that force air into the lungs when the patient has stopped breathing." So, when they have a hundred-year-old person with very advanced dementia, weighing seventy pounds, locked in a fetal position, and already in the active dying process, advocates of level one would surgically implant a tube in the patient's stomach to force food in and also put the electric paddles on the patient's chest to force the heart to start again. Of the physicians polled in this study, 1.6% agreed with using level one if necessary to prolong the life. That choice sounds to me like just doing anything to keep a heart beating. I can't help but question the logic or motives of a medical practitioner who would follow that agenda. Is that death with dignity? Not to my way of thinking. I know I wouldn't let anyone do that to my mother. Again, as I wrote earlier, make sure you have an Advance Directive filled out if you don't want to possibly end up in such a situation. And, try to find a primary care physician whom you can work with.

*****

Three months later Mother was reexamined per hospice regulations to see if she was still qualified to have the required diagnosis. Mother's health had improved enough that she had to be removed from hospice—she no longer met the time qualification. I was happy to see Bernice's health improved but sorry to see the removal of the extra hands-on care by hospice. The following month she declined again, so I was able to get her back in hospice. A month after that, there was a new emergency with Mother, and this one illustrates how wrongly things can go for patients unable to communicate.

Bear with me as I relate how a series of medical mistakes can be so easily made—

I was with Mother at the nursing home on a Saturday afternoon and noticed something wrong with her leg. After I told the nurse and she had looked at the leg, she said with some worry that it could be a blood clot. (Neither nurses nor aides had mentioned the clot or disfigurement.) The nurse then called Mother's doctor and left a message with the doctor's service. Having come to the nursing home from the gym, I told the nurse I was going home to clean up and would call back to check on what the doctor said.

Mother was enrolled in hospice at this time, and her doctor— who was also the principal hospice doctor—was out of town. The doctor's partner, the covering physician, said to send Mother to the Emergency Room, so they sent her in an ambulance with her medical records. Mistake #1—as a hospice patient, Bernice shouldn't have been automatically ordered by the covering physician to the ER for treatment.

At the ER, a clerk looked at Mother's computer record based on a previous admission, instead of the current written records that had been sent along with her in the ambulance. Then the clerk took the name of the doctor listed in the computer record, and called him to see what that doctor's orders were. Mistake #2—the clerk should have looked at the current, written records which were there and always accompanied patients from the nursing home. Mistake #3—the clerk called the wrong doctor—Mother's previous doctor—to see what his orders were.

So, hearing from the clerk at the ER, Mother's previous doctor said to admit Bernice and begin treatment. Mistake #4—this previous doctor didn't even know that Mother wasn't his patient anymore and hadn't been for awhile. Then, without further checking of her records, he ordered her hospitalized and treatment to begin.

While visiting Mother in the hospital later that day, I spoke with her nurse on the ward and found out about the curative treatment that shouldn't have begun, since Bernice was a hospice patient.

I notified the hospice nurse on call and told her of the series of mistakes leading to this treatment. She said, "If you allow this treatment to continue, you have to withdraw your mother from hospice. Once she returns to the nursing home, you can have her reexamined to see if she'll be accepted into hospice again."

That treatment was a mistake; however, since it had begun I didn't think I should stop it. I had a call in for the doctor who made that decision but hadn't heard back from him. I told the hospice nurse that I would allow the treatment to continue, and the hospice nurse came to the hospital later in the day to have me complete paperwork withdrawing Mother from hospice.

When I later spoke with Mother's previous physician, he admitted that he made those decisions without realizing Mother wasn't his patient anymore. He had received the call from the clerk at ER and didn't think to question the clerk further.

*****

In a few days, Mother was repaired once again to the point where she could be returned to the nursing home. Mother's doctor was back in town and came by to verify that Bernice was qualified to enter the hospice program again.

Bernice was conscious, smiling, and back in her wheelchair. She was back to her normal routine. I still found the sparkle in her eye, but she was very tired.

I had made it a point to tell Mother in these later years that it was okay if she wanted to leave. Further, that I would miss her a great deal, but I wanted most of all for her body to be at peace and her spirit to soar.

A couple of the nurses at the facility felt that Bernice had lived so long because she felt so loved—that the bond between the two of us kept her going. The nurses enjoyed watching her face light up when I got off the elevator, and we saw each other.

At the end of that month—February 2002—Mother got another infection. She was six weeks short of her 89th birthday.

The hospice nurse called to tell me what the options were: 1) Send Mother to the hospital for the most aggressive treatment against the infection and subsequently lose hospice again; 2) Treat her at the nursing home with a strong intramuscular antibiotic; or finally 3) Stick to palliative care and concentrate on her comfort.

The decision was up to me, and that meant there would be no error in the handling of her treatment this time. Considering all I knew of Mother and her wishes, I chose for her to stay at the nursing home and take the lesser antibiotics. In essence, that choice was much closer to palliative care than the other choice—aggressive, curative hospital treatment. That decision was a new direction. It was the first time that critical decision was made by me, and I felt the consequences as I made it.

*****

A couple of days later I received a call from a hospice nurse who was then at NH #3. She said that the antibiotics weren't working. At that point, I went to the nursing home to speak with the nurse in person. She then estimated Mother's remaining life to be seven days or less. I still had the option of choosing the aggressive hospital treatment and leaving hospice, but I said no. Mother was far too tired to suffer through the hospital treatment.

That was a stab of reality for me. Mother and I had been through so much over the last eleven years—all the ups and downs of the AD and concurrent illnesses—now the uncertainty of end date was gone. The time was upon us.

The first two nights I stayed with Mother until 3 AM and then went home to rest before going to work. The third day she was getting worse, and I decided to stay there from then on.

On the third night, March 7, 2002, her fever was climbing, and the Tylenol didn't seem to slow it down. She was also receiving some medication for "air hunger"—the rapid breathing due to low blood oxygen levels and cardiac stress.

After peaking at 102 degrees around 10 PM, her temperature did start lowering. Also, her blood pressure and pulse began to fall. It appeared that she would pass away that night.

Though unconscious, her face looked so relaxed, as though she had a "conscious peacefulness." There was no smile, just a relaxed countenance. The look reminded me of the face on the most common statue of the Buddha—detached peacefulness.

By 10 PM we were alone, just as we had spent so much time over those past eleven years. It was as it should have been—we had started this journey together long ago, and now the two of us were to complete it.

The finest person I had ever known, or known of, was about to pass away. As she had humbly set a model of how a good life is lived, she now calmly demonstrated how the inevitable end is graciously accepted. This joyful lady had so happily awaited the birth of her five children and loved them all so much from day one on through the end of her life. She had taught us all that life is to be enjoyed and to appreciate all the simple little things along the way; to be grateful for what we have; to have an optimistic and positive attitude; to help our fellow beings; to smile and laugh and love; and so much more.

Nurses came in at intervals to offer any assistance they could. They also brought in a tray with coffee and water. Out of consideration, they had moved out my mother's roommate; I had that bed available if I needed to rest.

Bernice was very popular with the nurses and CNAs due to her near-perpetual smile or laugh, the sparkle in her eye, and her habit of reaching out to help others—literally reaching out from her wheelchair when someone passed her who was in despair. No matter how advanced the AD became, it never diminished her compassion for suffering people.

The aides always enjoyed feeding her in the dining room because she had a good appetite and made their job easy. They would raise a spoon of food to her lips, and she would open her mouth to readily take it in, just like a baby. Some difficult residents would keep their mouth closed, or spit out the food once it was in their mouths. So, every aide or assisting nurse wanted the job of feeding Bernice.

Hospice assistance at this point was in the medications provided, and instruction given to Bernice's nurses on administering them. I know that Mother and I both appreciated that help very much.

About midnight, I told Mother again that I loved her, and I thanked her so much for being my mother. It was becoming harder and harder to hold the tears in, but thankfully there were as many of joy as of sadness. Those of sadness were for my loss; those of joy were for her much-deserved release.

I told her that I would be starting the flower and vegetable seeds soon, then moving the transplants to the garden, and of course I would need her help in the garden that summer. I had no doubt that her spirit would join me.

I looked at the wall by her bed and saw the large poster of butterflies Nancy and I had brought her five years earlier. The poster showed a variety of life-sized butterflies flying around a pink azalea bush, so happy and free. And I thought of her freedom so near at hand. She was so close to shedding the cocoon and spreading her wings.

My eyes moved to the wall at the foot of her bed. There hung the poster made from the photo of our foreheads together. That photo was a spontaneous shot taken five years earlier. My thought was that as verbal communication diminished, perhaps our brains could communicate through the foreheads touching. That's why I was chuckling in the photo.

I hung that poster at the foot of her bed, so that Mother could find some comfort whenever she awoke and found herself lost or disoriented. So many staff told me they loved that photo and especially the poster made from it.

At 2 AM, I whispered in her ear. "We've made it, Mother. We won." We definitely had won, and I wanted to share that with Mother before she was gone. As Bernice had dealt with the inner confusion and sense of loss resulting from AD, I kept the outer problems at bay. The disease never did break her spirit. Her sparkling smile and pattern of joyful love was evident until she slipped into unconsciousness.

I assured her again that whenever she felt ready, to feel free to leave. I spoke of loving her and appreciating what a great Mother and great person she had been throughout my life. Also, that living by good example, she had inspired love in a lot of other people.

Then I asked a final wish of her—that I could see her smile just one more time. At this time, she was breathing through her mouth with her lips forming an "O," and her eyes were still closed. Slowly I saw her cheeks widen as the corners of her mouth turned up a slight bit; and the "O" was making the beginning of an oval—a final smile. So I said, "Thank you, Mother" and kissed her on the forehead. From that, I knew that we were still in some conscious contact.

At 3:15 AM I said, "Mother, I have to lie down for a little while. I'll be in the other bed just a few feet away." Then I told the floor nurse who checked in regularly, "If anything changes, let me know." At 3:30 AM, Chuck shook me and said, "Heydon, she's leaving us." I took the two steps over to her bed, and she was gone.

She had just slowed down over the course of the night and was in no pain or distress or anxiety. Her blood pressure and respiration rate just slowed down until they stopped.

An RN came up from the first floor to do the final check for vital signs. At 3:35 AM, she told me what I already knew; she made it official with, "Heydon, I'm afraid I have to tell you she's not with us any longer."

I sat alone with her body for quite awhile and felt very much at peace, relaxing in the tranquility of the early morning before the sun came up. The peace seemed like a message from Mother saying "Thank you. All is well." It was late winter and a good time to die, allowing a couple of weeks before the resurrection of all human, animal and plant spirits in the spring.

A bright light went out on earth. A new angel arose in the heavens.

*****

As I remember, Lori—the other helpful nurse that night—called the funeral home. I had stayed with Mother for an hour and a half in the silence of the early winter morning before the driver arrived. He took her away at 5:40 AM.

Soon after Mother was taken away, I prepared to leave the nursing home myself. I saw Lori at the nurses' station, and I could see that she was affected by Bernice's passing as well. She said, "During nurses' training, they stress how important it is to control our emotions, but sometimes…sometimes, it's just so hard…" I thanked her for her help, and then I went out into the cold, winter air.

By the time I got home, the light of dawn was up, and a new day was beginning. I was exhausted and numbness had set in.

After a few hours of fitful sleep, I went to the funeral home with my wife and one of my sisters to make the final funeral arrangements. We had prepaid the funeral about ten years earlier; at this point, we planned the visitation, the burial service, providing the obituary, and going over any additional services we might need.

The double headstone was already in place from when we buried Dad eleven years earlier. The only missing portion was to add the engraving of Mother's date of death. The stone would read, "Heydon W. Buchanan, 1913-1991, Colonel, Infantry" and "Bernice I. Buchanan, 1913-2002, Beloved Wife."

✝✝✝✝

Visitation was set for two days later, on a Sunday afternoon. Friends and family stopped by to pay respects, and some to view her for a final time. At visitation, two people warned me before I saw Mother that it didn't really look like her. I checked the casket and agreed and further suggested we keep the casket closed during visitation. It was her mouth that seemed so different; I imagine the mouth is difficult for morticians to match when some or all of the teeth are missing. However, one sister was adamant that it did look like Mother and wanted to keep the casket open, so I quietly told her to do what she wanted. Visitation is certainly not the place to have disagreements.

As a visual review of her life, I placed twenty-four photos of her and various members of our family in a 3 x 2 foot frame and put it on a palette. With four rows of six photos each, the period went from a few weeks after her birth in 1913 through a photo of the two of us taken in 1997. That photo was taken by my wife and is truly a favorite of mine. I assembled this collection a couple of years earlier to hang in her room at the nursing home. The purpose was for the staff to see Bernice's whole life as opposed to only knowing her current condition as a resident.

*****

Funeral services were set for Monday morning. Bernice would be buried next to her husband in Crown Hill Cemetery, a very historic burial ground and the third or fourth largest cemetery in the United States. It was founded in 1864 as a burial ground for American Civil War soldiers—many Confederate prisoners of war (POWs) as well as Union troops.

Mother would be placed among so many of the heartland's citizens who had preceded her. All of them were surrounded and entwined by celebrated presences of the past—Veterans from the Civil War and subsequent wars and military service, and the more glorified and notorious citizens from James Whitcomb Riley to John Dillinger to Benjamin Harrison to Eli Lilly and on and on. Elegant and stoic mausoleums and obelisks among a sea of more simple horizontal and vertical stone markers—all of these are set in rolling woodlands with a few hills and a variety of beautiful, stately trees.

Each season I walk through Crown Hill with an old friend on our quarterly pilgrimage. We reflect on current and past events of our lives and families, and try to refresh our perspective on life. As we pass the grave markers, I can hear the voices of old souls as though from *Spoon River Anthology.*[2] "I was a poet," says one. "I was a bank robber," says another. "I was the President of the United States," says a third. "I was a pharmacist," says the fourth man.

Soon, our walks through history would have Mother's voice added to Dad's. Soon, I would hear Dad's greeting, "I was a soldier," joined by Bernice's, "I was a Mother and homemaker and a happy person."

Bernice would join so many other unsung heroines in the cemetery—ladies whose quiet and unspoken achievements made it possible for the men to receive the acclaim.

*****

As a service prior to burial, we had a memorial in a small gothic chapel set in the oldest portion of the cemetery. The chapel is a simple but stately old structure built of Indiana limestone. One can feel the history before even walking in the door. On entering, one seems to hear the echoes of so many farewells spoken by the living to the dead.

Children and grandchildren of Bernice took turns speaking to the assembled mourners about the qualities of this loved one who had just left us. One of my sisters spoke about how fair Mother was with all of us. Another spoke of how well she did as a homemaker, nourishing all of us daily.

Before I got up to speak, I turned to my wife and said, "I don't know if I'll be able to finish my comments. If I can't, would you finish this list for me?" And she said sure she would. However, I did make it through my talk. I spoke of Bernice's life and her ancestors. Her great-grandfather was one of the half dozen pioneers who settled the town of Tampico, Illinois. Her parents moved to Indiana with her dad's work in the lumber business. Then I spoke of Mother meeting Bud and making a very productive life together…the birth of their children…the challenges of the Depression and two wars for Dad…the happiness and joy of simple things and having each other. I added that she was a wonderful daughter, wife, mother, grandmother, friend and community member. She was much-loved by all who knew her.

I think most people wondered what was Bernice's secret—the secret to having such a sturdy supply of happiness and joy. For one thing, she accepted life on its own terms. She had very strong faith. I believe another part of it was in following the principles she had been taught at a young age. "Do unto others as you would have them do unto you." "If you can't say something nice, don't say anything at all."

Reflecting on this last principle, I'm reminded of a biography on Abraham Lincoln titled, *With malice toward none: the life of Abraham Lincoln.*[3] Like Abe, Mother did not feel malice toward anyone.

My wife Nancy was the final speaker. She chose to read a poem I had written for Mother twenty years earlier and included on a Mother's Day card. Mother and Dad had saved all the letters I had written from various parts of the country and the world. Also, Mother had saved all the Mother's Day cards I had sent.

So Nancy read—

Without a Mother who would be
Or see or hear or know of life.
The one who brought us to this world
And buffered us from pain and strife.

The extra care she always gives
Can always change our bad to good.
The extra ear she always has
Will often change our 'can't' to 'could.'

Our spirits always feel this force
While near at hand or far apart.
The knowing child will always say,
"I'm glad, Dear Mother, we share a heart."

After Nancy read this, I remembered that particular Mother's Day and calling her and Dad to say hello. After I had spoken with her,

Dad got on the phone, saying privately to me, "You sure made Mother happy today." Well, I was happy that I could do it.

Needless to say, so many parents make countless sacrifices for their children. However, in the case of mothers, the example can be truly awe-inspiring. As one tiny example of what they do, my mother always knew where every single piece of clothing was at any time for all six of us; and she knew the location of every book or toy or whatever. How she could do that by herself was beyond my comprehension. Maybe it's in a woman's genetic code to some degree. I say it's no wonder that she got dementia, as her mind was probably taxed out.

*****

So, the Memorial ended, and we drove the short distance to the burial plot. It was time to speak our final good-byes silently and lower the casket into the ground. Each child placed a rose on the casket and kneeled for a last thought. It was done.

After the service was over, I went to the office of the funeral home in order to settle some final details. I wanted to have a vase installed on Mother's & Dad's stone so I could bring them flowers from the summer garden. Also, I had an additional engraving done on Mother's side of the stone, which read "LOVING MOTHER."

Following that, I turned to the funeral director and thanked her for her help. I also noted that there weren't many people at the funeral compared to my father's burial, but that there weren't many people at the funeral of Jesus either.

She replied, "From what I heard as all of you spoke about her life, I thought you *were* talking about Jesus Christ." No matter what differences the offspring had had concerning caregiving and the subsequent struggles, each person realized the wonderful qualities of this person whom we had been fortunate enough to call Mother.

With the final details settled, we drove away, leaving the mortuary office and the cemetery, as well as the gravediggers who had to finish the final phase of their work.

I had attended a half dozen visitations and funerals of nursing home residents while Mother was at the nursing home. These deceased residents were friends and acquaintances I had known during those institution years. I had seen their family members at least several times a week during that period, and known them during my time on the Family

Council. We had struggled together, and then I helped say good-bye to their loved ones when they had passed away. Mother's funeral would be my last of the nursing home series.

While driving home, I kept thinking of this loss—as Mother, as teacher, as a model of what I imagine a great person to be. I was most fortunate to have this spiritual influence in my life. This was someone who walked in the Grace of God.

Even witnessing another's passing still doesn't bring the realization that that door is one through which we will all pass. Somehow, it's still hard for me to realize that someday I will be passing through that door. Ultimately, I believe that good things are in store.

*****

We arrived home and went indoors. I was somewhat amazed that I had made it through the last few days with few tears. From the moment Mother passed away until then, I had not given in to any mourning emotion; I thought I might at the memorial, but I had made it through. I was still in a type of numb shock. It was so hard to believe that she was gone. We had been through so much for so many years. The caregiving seemed like it would never finish. Following her burial, I felt the active caregiving had finally come to an end.

I looked at Nancy and started to say something. After opening my mouth, I felt something coming up through my throat. Then it all poured out—choking sobs that I hadn't felt since I was a child. I was finally able to cry.

CHAPTER 12

PICKING UP THE PIECES

Do not stand at my grave and weep. I am not there;
I do not sleep. I am a thousand winds that blow. I am
the diamond glint on snow. I am the gentle autumn rain.
I am the sun-ripened golden grain. And when you wake in
the morning hush, I am the swift uplifting rush of circling
birds and circling flight. I am the soft starlight at night.
Do not stand by my grave and weep. I am not there;
I do not sleep.
　—Navajo Epitaph

FOR AT LEAST SEVERAL YEARS BEFORE MOTHER'S PASSING, I HAD been preparing myself for the day, at least as much as I could prepare. Is anyone ever really ready for their loved one to pass away, especially their closest connection on Earth? In speaking with friends I would say, "I want her suffering to end, but I also know that I will miss her so much." On some level, I'm sure I wanted my own struggles to end as well, but that was truly a distant consideration, or at least a subconscious one.

I considered the phrases that I had heard with reference to death by Alzheimer's disease (AD). The first was "The long goodbye." The second was "The funeral that never ends." Both seemed appropriate, but the second one about the endless funeral better illustrates the continuing grief.

From different sources I hear people speak of mourning their AD patient throughout the disease and therefore they are numb at funeral time. I was somewhat numb when death actually occurred. However, my experience of mourning was different. During the disease, I just seemed constantly busy with handling the endless details of her care and trying to make her remaining time as pleasant as possible. Some caregivers mourn each day for the new portion of mental loss by their loved one. I celebrated each day the portion of Mother that remained. We could smile and laugh until near the end, and that made a difference in how I perceived her dying process.

Mother's final three days were when the reality of her approaching end finally hit home. The news was brief but powerful—"The antibiotic isn't working. She may have seven days left." That was a real marker, no more vague guesses. More striking to me was watching her enter into semi-consciousness and then begin slipping away from the world; it was watching her eyes close, and seeing her breathing through her mouth which was formed as a small circle. Seeing Mother in that state made me very aware not only of her approaching end but also of her recently-added diagnosis: cachexia—wasting away. Her body was so tired, and it was time. It wouldn't take a week to end—she had three days left.

Bernice had done her part in life for so long. She accepted the tough things that came her way, and she never complained. She set the model for accepting life as it came and God's plan whatever that may be. She had the inner strength of her faith, and the love it produced. She led a remarkable yet humble life, and she was ready to see her Maker. I had no doubt that God's greeting to her would be, "This is my daughter, of whom I am very proud."

I thought again of my comment to her in those last few hours—the mention of our victory. Now, all was done, for her anyway.

*****

Following the funeral, I had a few hours of fitful sleep. Then I got up but still couldn't think. My body was sore and restless. My mind was numb. I couldn't see the point of forcing myself to rest when it didn't help. My need then was to stress my body and balance my mind. I could think and rest better after that.

That evening I went to the gym to do a Step Aerobics class. As I went into the class I wasn't my normal smiling and upbeat self. Alicia, my instructor of many years, must have noticed and as she walked by me said, "We missed you on Saturday." Our regular Saturday morning class was a great way to begin the weekend.

"Yes," I replied, "I couldn't come. It was something serious."

"I hope it worked out okay," she said.

"No, it didn't," I answered. Then I walked over to where she was standing and told her what had happened.

"I'm so sorry for your loss." Alicia said very sincerely. "If she was anything like you, she must have been very special."

"Thanks, Alicia," I replied, "but she was worlds ahead of me." And that was an understatement.

Bernice Ione Foy Buchanan was the most phenomenal and outstanding human being I've known, or known of, during my life. She led a most exemplary life. Throughout my existence, and especially during my eleven years of caregiving, she continued to teach by example. She stayed strong and humble, true to her faith, honest with herself and all human beings, forever helpful, forever joyful, forever loving and compassionate.

A combination of people and events and inherent nature went into making this unique human being. Grandma Pet—the joyful heart of Tampico, Illinois, and the wellspring of Mother's laughter, was especially dedicated to Bernice, her only granddaughter, and taught her the delight of working with love.

Earlier this year, another resident of early Tampico passed away—Ronald Reagan. In that very small town, I have no doubt that he knew Grandma Pet, and may well have been influenced by her in a positive vein. In later years, Mr. Reagan referred to his second stay in Tampico—age seven to nine—as his "Huck Finn" period. The down-home, cheerful, and optimistic part of his nature was similar to Bernice's; however, with Mother, those positive traits were not just part of her nature but permeated her entire character, and always merged with the hard work she happily did, and the love she endlessly gave. Of course that purity is easier for a loving Mother to maintain than it would be for an actor and politician whose work requires a chameleon-like persona. I believe Mr. Reagan would agree with me on this. The point is that his common-folk, pioneer persona and charm were important in helping him get elected.

There is significance to time and place in the development of our lives. In the development of our country, no region is more prominently noted for heart, soul, and humility than the Midwest—the Heartland. Though the degree of those traits will vary with the period of its history, this region still maintains a good nurturing ground overall. The temptations and distractions are also here; however, if a person can stay focused, they will still find it a good environment in which to grow.

The above factors illustrate the foundation of this unique human being—Bernice Buchanan, someone who made a major difference in my life and that of others, as well as presenting a beacon of light to the world.

*****

When the numbness made way for reflection, I began to think of my new reality—life after long-term caregiving, life without Mother, life without my closest friend, life without a consuming sense of purpose, and on, and on.

Mother and I were kindred spirits. It was not just the Mother-Son relationship, nor even the long years of caregiving that had bonded us yet stronger. As her dementia increased, we moved from Mother-Son to good friends, then to my making the necessary decisions and taking full responsibility for her welfare. Finally, there was a return to our most basic of natures—two friendly souls who always enjoyed each other's company, and who understood and appreciated the value of simple laughter and love in the human condition.

In current discussions on AD caregiving, there is much reference to role reversal as an adult child assumes the parental role while the parent becomes the child. The idea or implication is that the role switch is made one time, when the patient reaches a certain level of dementia.

My experience was a bit different from that on two counts. First, I found the disease to change in an inconsistent pattern; that is, instead of moving steadily downward, Mother went two steps down and then one back up. She was going progressively downward but the pattern was in stops and stutters instead of a steady angle decline. So that meant I wanted to be flexible in taking the reins when necessary and then giving control back to her when she was willing and able. The switch in control was subtle, and the average person probably wouldn't have noticed it.

The whole point of that style was to give her as much dignity as possible, and yet provide the support she needed when conditions overwhelmed her—the lower the stress, the calmer the mind was my thinking. I saw that method as not only giving her better mental and emotional health but subsequently slowing the progression of the disease. At least I felt it did, though it is difficult to qualify or quantify. Mainly, that process was based on keeping her as comfortable as possible in all respects. I considered it what I would want a caregiver to do for me if I were in that condition.

*****

While reflecting on Bernice's demeanor, I was reminded of a scene on the news a few years ago. The Dalai Lama was visiting the United States and greeting followers and well-wishers. As he stepped out of his car, an old couple smiled and bowed to him, and he returned the recognition. Both he and the couple were smiling and giggling a bit. Those actions probably helped overcome some awkwardness caused by the language barrier and also demonstrated good feelings and intent. Smiles and laughter are often the international signs of welcome.

That scene of the Dalai Lama reminded me so much of Mother and the way she often greeted people, especially as her mind faded and a language barrier came about, just like that of the Dalai Lama and the elder Americans. It was as though Bernice and the Dalai Lama were nurtured by the same Masters, either before or during this life.

Bernice Buchanan was always welcoming and of good intent to other people. Her sparkling smile and pattern of joyful love were evident until she slipped into semi-consciousness three days before passing away. Then her face took on a more tranquil demeanor—some combination of being serene and non-committal or detached, like the common pose of the Buddha.

*****

The loss of one's mother is hard; the loss of a great mother even harder; the loss of a great friend, yet more. The loss of a great humanitarian— well, that is society's loss. I know that it is better for her now. I keep telling myself that, but for me there's still an overriding sense of emptiness. I have appreciated the thrill of her victory; hopefully, when I finish writing this account of our journey, I'll move on to the joy of mine.

It is only now that I'm beginning to realize that my caregiving/guardianship of Mother is over. From January 12, 1991, when I first made the commitment to help her through this affliction, until March 11, 2002, when we buried her, my primary focus was always on her welfare. From the moment my eyes opened in the morning until they closed at night, her well-being was my number one concern. Those eleven plus years were very intense.

I have no regrets concerning my choice to watch over her. She spent her life giving to others and never asked anything for herself. She had a gentle dignity, full integrity and large amounts of joy and love. She raised five children and a demanding husband, and still stayed as calm as could be. Bernice Buchanan was unique, and I believe she walked in the Grace of God.

The bottom line may simply be that Bernice lived a full life and set a great example for the rest of us to follow. I know that that will be my challenge day after day—to incorporate more of those traits into my life, to feel that joyful acceptance deep into the soul until you realize that that is Enlightenment.

The 1990s in the United States were about financial investments. From every direction and medium, there was constant barking about which financial vehicle to put one's money in. The stock market kept rising, as well as any number of other markets, and a great deal of money was made.

I—like many other primary and solitary caregivers—heard a different drummer and subsequently made investments in the spiritual realm. My financial assets—very modest at best—fell during the 90s; half were used to fund my caregiving. My spiritual assets rose and fell during that period, depending on the challenge or crisis at hand.

My heart-and-soul investment in caregiving was similar in effect to the Japanese style of financial investments— thinking long-term; expecting, or at least willing, to take losses for quite awhile; yet believing in long-term rewards.

In the end, my spiritual assets began to rise consistently. To borrow the words of an ancient wise man, "Build up your treasures in heaven where they won't rust, and thieves can't break in and steal them." That made sense to me, and it still does. Caregiving for a loved one was the key to those spiritual dividends. The years, intensity, love, and sincerity of the caregiving were the deposits and measure of that account.

During the long, rocky climb of caregiving, I sometimes pondered whether I was doing the right thing by one choice or another. I got so tired that it was sometimes hard to think straight. More often, I wondered if I had the resources—financial, mental, physical, emotional, and spiritual—to complete this commitment I had made. The caregiving lasted eleven years—more than twice the amount of time I had guessed at the beginning.

Any doubt I had about the tasks and my capacity to do them didn't last long. Seeing a smile on Mother's face and the sparkle in her eye would quickly dissipate any doubts. There was no question that I was doing the most important thing I could be doing on earth. If I were to face my death at that moment, I wouldn't have been sad or regretful. Good things are generally expensive. The best can cost you years and years, if not your life.

*****

The day of Mother's burial drew to a close. I sat alone that night and wrote the following poem—

> As the darkness of this night arrived,
> I felt not only the end of the day
> But much, much more—
> The end of a life,
> The loss of my best friend,
> And most beloved symbol of joy.
> The last view of the body
> That brought me into this world,
> The body and soul that delivered,
>   nurtured and guided me,
> When I was at ease long enough
>   to absorb the lessons.
> The soul left my sight three days ago.
> The body now follows.

I cry for my loss.
My body convulses from the dreadful hurt
      that is bound to leave slowly.

I cheer for her victory.
Never faltering, she embraced
      truth, joy and love early in life.
Then she shared them with her family,
And all who came into contact with her.
As a wholesome example, she lived the lessons
      and also taught us.
She was much-loved and admired by all who knew her.

A bright light has left the earth.
A new angel has brightened the heavens.

Today brought another end,
That of my primary commitment to her welfare
      started more than eleven years past;
The commitment above all to her well-being
As the darkness of dementia began to chip away
      at her memory and other faculties.
Yet the dreaded disease could not conquer
      her loving and cheerful countenance.
Her complete alignment with a loving God
Earned her a rare exclusion from the
      standard frenetic human life.
As her body was lowered into the earth,
My daily priority of her well-being
      came to an end.

Today brought yet another end—
The completion of a promise to my father
      that I would take care of Mother until the end.
This agreement was secondary, though consistent
      with the promise I made to her.

Right before her passing,
I whispered in her ear,
"We've made it, Mother. We've made it!"

"Peace be with you until we meet again."
Soon after, she drifted away.

It's two minutes to midnight.
Everything now ends.
I drift off to sleep
And blanket myself with
          the love and joy she gave us all.

*****

Two days after Mother passed away, I returned to her room at NH #3 to start taking her things home. The transport took a few trips and was spread over two days. Some family members have difficulty in returning to the nursing home after their loved one's death. My sister was such a person as I could tell when she later thanked me for doing that task. I didn't have such trouble in going back. Perhaps I was still numb from the death, and that accounted for part of it. However, there were a couple of more important reasons. First, Bernice was now free, and I felt some joy that her suffering was over. Secondly, I never thought of the nursing home as being Mother's home, nor really had I thought of her as a permanent resident there. She was there over six years, but I thought of it as a medical service where she was in transit. She had left her real home to temporarily stay in the nursing facility before moving on to her better, well-deserved home.

Several days after the funeral, we bought a nice meal for all the staff at NH #3. It could be heated up in their kitchen ovens and provided during the day and evening as the working schedule permitted. It was a gift of thanks and was much appreciated. Many of the staff spoke of enjoying the photo of Mother and me that covers this book, so I made reprints and handed them out.

*****

About two weeks after Mother passed away, I turned on a TV for some distraction. The first scene was a flock of penguins rocking from side to side and smiling for the cameras. Then I realized it was the Academy Awards night. On the scale of importance, I couldn't help but think how empty and meaningless that whole scene was. There was this large group of overpaid, pampered movie stars having an exclusive costume party and trying to appear meaningful as they began another self-congratulatory celebration. I love a good story and one that has been dramatized by a cohesive group of skilled actors and support crew; however, these things need to be kept in perspective. People in the filmmaking business seem to live in the land of fairy tales.

I thought about the unsung heroes and heroines of everyday life who sacrifice much and receive little in recognition. I thought about the significance of the life and death of a loved one—a great soul. So, I quickly turned the TV off and went back to dealing with reality. I needed to begin incorporating this loss into my soul and not veer off into escapism.

The day after that TV experience, I received a phone call from Susan—the bereavement director at the hospice service we used. The hospice personnel I had worked with were very compassionate, and Susan was especially so. Her branch of the service would probably require that, and her background as a social worker helped.

Susan gave me a briefing on the bereavement services and asked if I would like to speak with someone concerning my loss. She was also very accommodating about where and when I might want to meet—her office or our home or wherever or whenever. She came to our home soon after. We spoke for a little while, and she left a couple of books.

Bereavement—or grieving—service is available to family members of the hospice patient for a year or more after the death. One of their services is group meetings for survivors to discuss their loss/losses and how they are coping now. The group sessions are two hours long, meeting weekly for six weeks. Another service is to be available for survivors who individually need to speak with someone about the death of their loved one or the death process. They also have a monthly news flyer with group schedules, some thoughts from the hospice chaplain, and prose or poetry by people who have been through their own loss.

I didn't feel a compelling need to go to a workshop, but I wanted to go. The first couple of groups had schedules during the day, so it interfered with work, and I couldn't make it. Then one gathering had an early evening schedule, and I signed up.

My group had six to eight people. There were many circumstantial differences, but we all blended very well. Our common bond was the recent loss of a loved one. As I remember, the differences were: 1) I was the only son; 2) the only male; 3) a bit younger than the rest; and 4) the only member who had lost someone to Alzheimer's disease. The ladies were all widows; some had remarried. It was a broad spectrum economically, and that was good. Two of the ladies had multiple deaths close together—a husband and a son, a husband and a daughter. Susan facilitated the group, and she had a hospice volunteer to help out.

Our first session included a "Welcome to the group"; a note on confidentiality; making out a "Grief report card" (how we were coping); respecting each other's grief and loss; support systems; and what I considered a very important point—the degree and duration of individual loss.

I noticed that I wasn't really grieving as the others were. Part of that may have been from the different relationships we all had with those who had died. Also, there was the matter of having left things unsaid for some, as their loved one had died suddenly. I had left nothing unsaid; felt that I had done all I could in caregiving; and found myself celebrating our journey and Mother's character more than anything else. I believe that positive note turned out to be helpful to some others in the group. Tears still came easily to my eyes, but they weren't generated by sadness so much as the sense of our victory.

The second session covered how we individually responded to loss and compared it to other losses in our lives. Also, there was a brief exercise in which we listed fifteen feelings we had about the death of our loved one. I had a wide range of feelings. My first fifteen were loss, pain, reward, wonder, joy, satisfaction, curiosity, disbelief, sadness, emptiness, acceptance, sorrow, love, confusion, and reality.

The third session covered myths about grief and something we'd done since the loss of our loved one that we were proud of. The thing I was proud of that I had done was cried; I had been thinking for years and years that I needed to cry, but the tears didn't come until after the funeral.

The fourth session involved taking care of ourselves. Also, there was the consideration of unfinished business—what we left unsaid and undone with our loved one. Finally, there was the matter of forgiving ourselves.

The fifth session involved a discussion of changing relationships, understanding the tasks of mourning and the journey of grief, and writing a letter to our loved one. I enjoyed the exercise of writing the letter. I still felt Mother's happiness and laughter, so writing a letter was not uncomfortable at all.

The final session included another self-evaluation on how we were coping with grieving, and making sure we controlled our own grieving without being pressured by others; that is, not letting anyone else tell us how long grieving should last.

During the course, we were asked to bring in a photo of our loved one if we so chose. I was happy to do so and brought in the same photo as is on the cover of this book. Everyone liked it, and the joyful communion it represented.

As I mentioned earlier, my sense of loss and my experience in the dying process were different from the other people in the class. I felt some joy mixed in with my loss, and I believe that brought light relief to the atmosphere—a counterweight. So my benefits from the class were different as well. A principal benefit for me was being able to share the positive side of what Mother and I went through.

One of the main discussions in that class was something I had considered well before attending the group. That was the big issue of defining personal grief. Perhaps that was because I had to face the matter somewhat during my caregiving; and even AD caregivers will vary in their grieving according to their individual circumstances.

Grieving Schedule and Duration

The schedule of grieving the loss of a loved one with Alzheimer's is as irregular and individual as the beginning and advancing of the disease itself. There is the matter of how close the survivor was to the patient with Alzheimer's. Was it a caregiver who lived with the victim and the disease day in and day out, or was it a relative or friend who may or may not have visited the patient occasionally? Was it a sensitive person who recognized and mourned the loss of their loved one, or was it someone more businesslike who dismissed the death quickly?

In my case, there was also the matter of mourning the loss of the family as I had known it—not only the passing of the second parent, but the damaged sibling relationships. This was a secondary loss that came about as a result of the disease, or at least how some people chose to respond to the disease. These relationships could be reconstituted in a new and agreeable style, but the previous open-ended trust and love would be very slow in returning.

Shortly after the funeral, one of my siblings said, "Mother was gone to me six or seven years ago." I'm not sure what determined her choice of the "goodbye" date. It may have been when a certain level of dementia was reached. Or, it may have resulted from not being involved with Mother's care, seeing very little of her, and finding it convenient to detach herself from the whole caregiving process.

Bernice's oldest friend in Indianapolis approached Mother's illness in another form of detachment. I called Selma occasionally to check on her health, as she was a widow and alone. She would always ask about Mother and how she was doing at the nursing home. At one point she said, "Heydon, I went to the nursing home to visit her once. While I was talking to her, she suddenly just turned her wheelchair around and started scooting down the hall. I don't think she knew who I was. I just couldn't go again." Another possibility for Selma's discomfort may have been that she was close to Mother's age and fearful of the nursing home awaiting her. So, Selma had her own way of grieving, or avoiding it.

Grieving is an individual process, and the style and duration of that event are simply based on the connection and understanding you shared with the person who passed away.

*****

The hospice had a candlelight Memorial Ceremony in December—nine months after Mother had passed away. About a hundred people were there to remember their loved ones. Each person held a lit candle and said a few words, if they chose, about their loved one who had passed away. It was very moving to see the room filled with only candle light, and so many people in common, respectful purpose—honoring their loved ones.

At the ceremony, I ran into Susan—the hospice bereavement director. She asked if I would be interested in speaking to a college class she was to teach in the spring. The students were seniors in social work and getting ready for graduate school, or to go right out into the world in their chosen vocation. Susan considered my caregiving situation very special and felt the students could benefit by my talk. I was happy to do so and agreed to give the talk.

In early April 2003, I spoke to her class. The scheduled forty-five minute talk including a question-and-answer session was still going strong after ninety minutes. The students were very interested in my experience and gave rapt attention; and that felt rewarding to me. After the talk, they asked a number of very perceptive and insightful questions. In a phrase, they were totally into it. As Susan walked me out afterwards, she thanked me a great deal for coming in and sharing my story. As a final word, she said, "Heydon, you're mesmerizing. You should do this for a living." As I walked to my truck, I thought, "I wish I could." The week after my talk, the class of about twenty-five students sent me a thank you card; everyone had signed it, and most wrote a little note as well. They were moved.

That experience really emphasized to me the therapeutic value of sharing such a powerful experience. It became part of my mourning process to speak with other people about caregiving for an AD patient; this was true when speaking one-on-one, and also in speaking to groups. The real emphasis in my talks has been about the value of love and acceptance in caregiving.

Soon after the university talk, I thought to do more talks on the subject if there was a need in the community. I spoke with the Education Director of the Alzheimer's Association in Indianapolis, and she asked me to consider being on their Speaker's Bureau. I happily agreed to speak for them when my schedule permitted.

The first talk Kate asked me to give for the Association in Indianapolis was a talk on grieving to a group of family members and survivors of a loved one who passed away from AD. My scheduled thirty-minute talk was expanded to an hour and a half when the bereavement director of a local hospice cancelled out on their portion at the last moment; as a result, our Q&A portion involved a lot of questions and discussion.

I felt very comfortable with the talk and answering questions until someone asked me, "How do you grieve for the passing of your care recipient if you didn't really like that person?" I was at a loss for an answer and so admitted, since I was very close to my care recipient and loved her greatly. Grieving and mourning are really individual matters in that they relate to a personal perception of the loss involved. The points

I shared with the group were the experiences of a longtime primary caregiver who was always very close to the care recipient.

Some caregivers and relatives speak of grieving the loss of their AD victim during the lengthy disease; that is, losing the loved one piece by piece and grieving that loss accordingly. I never felt that way, at least not consciously. I was far too busy trying to monitor her care; and, each day I celebrated the part of her mind that remained, as opposed to mourning the part which was gone.

An important thing to remember in terms of AD patients losing their faculties is that it doesn't usually happen suddenly and permanently. For example, your loved one may not recognize you one moment but a few minutes later they do recognize you. This pattern can continue until they don't recognize you at all. I define it as a very irregular pattern of loss. It is a progressive loss but also incremental—down two steps, back up one. Then the patient may stay on that step plateau for awhile. In an extreme condition of shock and stress, the patient can drop a long way in abilities; however, when rested, they can recoup much of that loss. This was the case I described in chapter seven about the Catastrophic Effect.

Throughout my caregiving, I felt as close to Mother as always. That increased her comfort level and most likely slowed the progression of her disease. We enjoyed each other's company to the end.

One of my primary goals was to show her that she was loved a great deal. Unlike many of the unfortunate residents who had no visitors and who often looked so forlorn, Mother received constant reinforcement of my feelings for her. Some residents would look at us with smiles; some would look with sadness as if to ask "Why couldn't that be me?" And a few would look on with jealousy. I would talk to the lonely ones and give them a pat on the shoulder. That would at least serve as a quick fix to their otherwise sad demeanor. Several of the long-term nurses at NH #3 felt that Bernice lived so long because she felt so loved.

As the years passed, there were times when I wished Mother's suffering could end—primarily for her but also for me. However, regardless of when she passed away, I knew that I would miss her terribly. I was always conscious of that. Such truly exceptional people do not often come along in one's life.

*****

When Mother had three days of life remaining, a new sadness came over me though I didn't think of it as grief. It was a shock to be faced with such definite news after so many years of intense caregiving with no end in sight.

On her final night of life, I stayed next to her and talked of our years together during this period and our victory over everything. I did not grieve then. After she passed away in the wee hours of the morning, I stayed by her side for a while. I was happy for her that it was done. I didn't grieve then either.

The grieving episode right after the funeral didn't last too long. However, I was on the verge of tears for a week. Even months after that when I spoke of her it was not difficult to feel some tears near by. Although I felt the loss of her physical presence quite strongly, I didn't feel any guilt or regrets. What I did feel was grateful to God that I stayed strong enough to last the eleven years of caregiving.

*****

What I learned, or relearned, during this whole experience was how individual the process of grieving can be. For intensity and length, grieving can only be defined by the individual. It cannot be qualified nor quantified by anyone else. No one can realize how much or how little another person hurts. No one can tell how long grieving will go on for another human.

People like systems—a set of understood rules to reduce things to black and white issues. Business especially desires systems, some standardized *quid pro quo*. In terms of the loss of a loved one, a business may give you three paid days off work for the loss of a spouse or child; two days off for the loss of a parent; and one day off for the loss of a grandparent. This may not be the amount for most businesses—if they give paid time off at all—but it does illustrate the hierarchical system to place a certain value on the loss of a loved one.

In another effort to systematize, some people think they can gauge a person's loss by the age of the person who died; that is, if the loved one you lost is elderly, someone might say, "Well, they were close to the end, anyway." or "They're really better off now." The person saying that may think they are comforting you. Someone made a similar comment to me a week or two after Mother passed away. Essentially, the comment was that while the disease had been long and drawn out, now Mother had passed away and things would probably return to normal soon; in essence, the mourning would be short.

I replied that it was quite a loss, regardless of the length of the illness. The intensity of long-term caregiving for a kindred spirit, in addition to the Mother-child/Mother-son relationship, made it a very strong connection. Making an analogy, I said that it would probably be similar to her losing her child. She was shocked and said, "Oh, no. Losing a child is not the same thing. You can't imagine that since you don't have children." I think she meant well in offering condolences, but she couldn't comprehend that what matters in loss is the significance of the deceased to the survivor, not the order of blood relationship. Spiritual loss is the only true barometer and really that can't be measured.

The only thing my acquaintance was truly saying was that for her to lose her mother would be much less grievous than if she lost her child. So, the reality is that her opinion of loss only applies to her life.

To draw on the common example of losing children, let me try another explanation. Let's say couple number one has four children while couple number two has one child. All of the children are involved in a plane crash. The first couple loses three of their children while the second couple suffers the loss of their only child. Which couple has suffered the greatest loss? We simply can't systematize or measure another person's loss and grief—not the depth, nor the intensity, nor the duration. Even two siblings losing the same parent grieve differently. That would appear as equal loss, but the reality of each sibling's loss and subsequent grief can be extremely different.

I'll offer one more scenario of two examples of loss. A man's wife dies, and he is so distraught that he takes his own life, leaving a note that reads "I cannot live without her." The second case is a parent losing a child to death, and the parent says, "My heart is broken at this loss. I will continue living, but I will never be the same." Which person has suffered the greatest loss? How do we gauge the depth of a person's pain? Simply put, no one can measure another's loss—neither by a set equation, nor by comparing it with their own.

In offering condolences, perhaps the only accurate and appropriate statement we can make is, "I'm sorry for your loss." Although we may think and say something to the contrary, in truth we don't know how they feel. We may remember how we felt when we lost a family member or friend, but each person's pain or perception of pain is based on his or her own uniqueness.

Concerning my experience, the loss of my mother—Bernice Buchanan—was the most major of losses. As Mother, friend, consultant, joyful community member and humble, exemplary member of her faith, she was without equal.

When mothers were being handed out, I believe God said, "Heydon, you need a good teacher—one who teaches by example with joy and love—or you will get way out of hand. Your father can guide you in certain ways, but serenity is not his forte. So, Bernice will be your ultimate guru for that calmness in action, and some day you will realize that."

*****

When I made the caregiving commitment, I had absolutely no idea of what would be happening—not in the short term, nor in the long run. My life was changed forever. This span of well over fifteen years—from my father's death and my commitment, until the end of this writing—has been the most significant period in my life.

The events, feelings, and radical changes made on the family and on the individuals involved were nothing short of truly revolutionary. In that vein, Mr. Dickens wrote in *A Tale of Two Cities'*—an account of the French Revolution—"It was the best of times. It was the worst of times." His opening lines seem to say it all.

I truly don't regret the decision I made, but I doubt if I could do it all over again at this point in my life, at least not to include all the outside problems Mother and I faced. The combination stressors of the Alzheimer's patient's needs plus the caregiver's needs plus that lingering sibling conflict plus nursing homes plus some of the aides and medical staff made for an incredible amount of stress—especially when it went on for over eleven years. In some respects, my caregiving experience was like going through the army—I wouldn't trade the experience for anything; but I don't think I could do it all again.

It is over now, but the effect on my life will be marked forever. Life will never be the same, nor should it be, for this is the essence of life—helping another human who is deeply in need. By the Grace of God, we made it through. Now I carry just memories of our victory.

When all is said and done, I will probably feel the loss of Mother's physical presence until my last day on earth. More importantly, I will feel her joy and love that long as well. In my mind, I can instantly see her lively smile and friendly prodding as she now says, "Let's go! Get on with life!"

CHAPTER 13

THE FUTURE— ALZHEIMER'S, NURSING HOMES, FAMILY CAREGIVING, AND ME

Those who love deeply never grow old; they may die of old age, but they die young.
  —Benjamin Franklin

Men are what their mothers made them.
  —Ralph Waldo Emerson

Arriving at one goal is the starting point to another.
  —Fyodor Dostoyevsky

For now, the best therapeutic tools we have for treating Alzheimer's disease are conscientious caregivers. By far, the best medication we have is love.
  —H.B.

S O NOW THIS JOURNEY ENDS, AND SO ENDS A MAJOR AND DEFINING portion of my life. Once this writing is over, I can relegate the subject to a more inactive portion of my mind—a place where disease and disability are overshadowed by the simple joys of living. I will continue to give talks on the caregiving experience for the Alzheimer's Association and other groups, but the dynamics of the disease will no longer have me in its grasp.

I'm beginning to see a life beyond the challenges of my last fifteen years—the eleven years of caregiving plus four years of lingering and compelling need to tell the story. Before stepping into my new life, I want to share some of my opinions and speculations on the future of the disease and nursing homes as well as aging and death in America. All of those subjects are related and intertwined.

Alzheimer's Disease and Caregiving

The present reality is that Alzheimer's disease (AD) controls us more than we control it. Very little has been discovered about its causes. At the time of this writing, current medications cannot stop it, reverse it, or even slow it down. And, they are of questionable value in even masking the progression of the disease as was reported at a recent major medical conference on the subject.[1] Patients and caregivers are desperate for some medical assistance, but there's not much in the way of hope that their doctor can provide. When pressed, the physician may prescribe something to try and temporarily help recall, but the doctors aren't seriously optimistic; they provide a sprig of hope for desperate AD patients and caregivers.

The above-referenced conference for doctors and other health care professionals was held at Johns Hopkins University in March 2004. The purpose was to discuss the value of current AD medications and other potential medical treatments for the disease. Perhaps the most telling remark of the gathering was given by Dr. Constantine G. Lyketsos, the Clinical Core Leader at The Johns Hopkins Alzheimer's Disease Research Center. He reportedly said, "The public thinks a cure is around the corner," but he doesn't expect any "realistic reduction in the huge number of cases for decades." His sentiments were echoed by other researchers at the conference as well.[2]

A recent PBS special production, *The Forgetting*,[3] based on the book of the same name by David Shenk,[4] covered the subject of AD and the catastrophic path we're on if we don't eliminate it. According to Mr. Shenk,[5] AD currently costs the nation about $100 billion annually; that is, lost income from patients who have to give up their jobs; lost income of caregivers who give up their jobs to take care of the patients; and the medical expenses of treating AD. Dr. Rudolph Tanzi is a neurogeneticist and one of the experts in the PBS show *The Forgetting*; he stated that with the addition of the babyboomer AD patients, and without any progress in treating the disease, by the year 2030 the entire federal budget will be spent on treating Alzheimer's disease.[6]

So, a very knowledgeable AD professional and other researchers have told us they don't expect any realistic reduction in AD patient numbers for decades; another told us that without progress in reducing the number of AD patients, the entire federal budget will be spent on AD treatment by the year 2030. As I write, it is the year 2006, so on our present course we're twenty-four years away from catastrophic disaster. That's pretty serious. If the U.S. government had decided to attack Alzheimer's disease instead of Iraq, perhaps we could have made some real progress by now in terms of slowing the onset and/or progression of the disease. Instead, we press on toward the Alzheimer's catastrophe so reasonably-predicted by the experts in the field.

*****

For now, the best therapeutic tools we have for treating Alzheimer's disease are conscientious caregivers. By far, the best medication we have is love. Those two aids may always remain as the most effective and powerful treatments in managing the disease. How we treat Alzheimer's patients is a pretty good measure of our own humanity—how we care for the vulnerable and defenseless members of our society who can't express their needs, grow weaker and more confused every day, and look to the rest of us to save them.

In 1996, a medical research study was published concerning older folks' attitudes toward receiving a diagnosis of Alzheimer's disease.[7] While 91.7% of the study participants would want to know if they had terminal cancer, only 79.5% would want to know if they had AD. Moreover, with a terminal cancer diagnosis, 80.2% of the participants would want their spouse to know of the diagnosis. With an AD diagnosis, only 65.7% of that group would want their spouse to know their diagnosis. One of the reasons given for wanting to know the AD diagnosis was *being able to consider suicide*. Needless to say, physicians have their hands full in trying to decide the best way to deliver such a diagnosis, or not to deliver it. The patient does have the option of not knowing his or her diagnosis if he or she chooses. Also, the patient has the right to not have his or her spouse or other family be told the diagnosis. Also, the patient has the right not to be tested for AD. Some patients have stated that they don't want to be tested for dementia. This last choice creates a new area for consideration— to determine exactly why those patients don't want to be tested.

An expansion of the 1996 study was published in 2003 with different results.[8] In the 2003 study, 92% of the subjects would want to know of an AD diagnosis while 86.5% would want to know about a terminal cancer diagnosis. While there were various reasons given for people wanting to know an AD diagnosis, the reason that 1.7% of the participants gave was that they *would consider suicide*. So, there is another challenge for the doctors to consider when delivering the AD diagnosis. One final note on that 2003 study is that participants with personal AD experience were significantly less likely to want to know if they had an AD diagnosis. The whole matter of delivering an AD diagnosis is complex to say the least.

It's interesting to see the mention of suicide by the respondents in the above two research studies. In the 1996 study, some participants would want to know if they had an AD diagnosis so they could *be able to consider suicide*. In the 2003 study, some participants faced with the same circumstances said they *would consider suicide*. My mother would never have considered suicide, and I'm happy that she didn't. However, I can't fault other people who have different considerations.

I don't believe the brief report I've given on those studies provides us with enough information to interpret the respondents' choices. Yet, it appears to reflect how seriously people consider and fear the disease and its consequences. For those subjects not wanting to know if they have the disease, those subjects not wanting their spouses to know if the subjects have the disease, and the smaller number of subjects who would consider suicide, I think of two possibilities for their replies: 1) a fear of the predictable Alzheimer's decline and death; and 2) a fear of being abandoned by his or her spouse on hearing that the subject has been diagnosed with AD. Those two thoughts are my first impressions. Regardless of any official study conclusion for the subjects' responses, I don't believe anyone would question the dire seriousness with which most people would receive the diagnosis of Alzheimer's disease.

*****

I should add a note on Alzheimer's disease and genetics, at least as I understand the subject with current research available. Having a parent with regular/late-onset Alzheimer's disease may increase a per-son's susceptibility to inheriting AD. However, there is no direct genetic link. Also, people without a genetic connection to AD get the disease as well. I reference late-onset AD above because the heredity factor is quite different with early-onset AD. That form of AD is rare but does have a direct genetic link. Moreover, early-onset AD strikes earlier in a person's life and progresses much faster, according to experienced caregivers. While I am accustomed to seeing and being around many AD patients after so many years of caregiving and visits to the nursing homes, I don't feel the same ease in the matter of early-onset Alzheimer's disease. That form of AD is truly a horror, and I have a special compassion for fami-lies afflicted with it. By striking people at a younger age, early-onset AD cuts short the working life of the victim and thereby affects the stability of a younger family which, for one thing, has more financial obligations for school-age children.

Nowadays, people of all ages are concerned about getting de-mentia. At least that's been my experience as so many people talk with me about it. Until Mother passed away, people would ask, "Are you worried about getting Alzheimer's since your Mother has it?" My reply was always the same, "No, I have enough concerns in daily life to keep me busy and free of that worry." And that was, and is, quite true. There is simply no point in dwelling on such a thing. I tell people not to worry about getting dementia or AD, to just do their best in life, take care of their health, and be optimistic as much as possible. After you've done your best, what will be, will be. If there is a marker in my genetic code to get AD, there's nothing I can do about that. As the street sage I refer-enced earlier said, "What is, is."

*****

With the continued rapid growth in the number of AD victims, no family in the country can remain untouched by the devastation. It is in everyone's interest to contemplate what you want if the disease should strike you, and to consider what you're willing to do to help a family member who may become an AD patient.

If you have an afflicted parent and want to help, ask what he or she would like in terms of help. Act quickly on the request. As soon as a diagnosis is received, have a family meeting with your siblings and the patient's spouse, if he or she is surviving and healthy. Discuss the diagnosis: what it means now and for the future; what the patient wants; what each person at the meeting is willing to give of themselves to achieve that; and also what other suggestions people at the meeting have with regard to treatment and caregiving.

Most importantly, conduct the meeting without emotion. Getting emotional during such an important discussion does not help anyone. The matter of handling this disease brings up intense feelings for all concerned. Too often, those emotions among siblings are volatile and act as a catalyst to divide people. In general, negative emotions are often expressed in an effort to intimidate other people, either consciously or unconsciously; there is no room for such nonsense in a serious meeting. The atmosphere of such a meeting should be in line with the respect required in a courtroom. If a family member is not mature enough to abide by those conditions, then he or she should not be allowed in the discussion. Expressing negative emotions is quite counterproductive in this situation and just serves to alienate people and set the discussion farther behind in finding a resolution.

If necessary, bring in an outside arbitrator to conduct the meeting. It could be a clergyman or social worker or therapist or doctor— someone that is acceptable to everyone at the meeting. The arbitrator would be independent of the family dynamics and able to keep the meeting on track toward developing an effective care plan. If an emotionally-controlled family member cannot peacefully participate in the family meeting; if that family member won't agree to having an arbitrator; if that family member can't tell at least one other family member what he or she is willing to do to help with caregiving for the afflicted parent; then I believe that troubled family member should be disregarded entirely in the matter of caregiving and not allowed at the meeting.

There is also the matter of family members who live at a great distance from the afflicted parent. That often ends up as a divisive factor among siblings for one reason or another, probably non-participation in caregiving by the distant member. I believe that there are ways for the sibling living far away to participate. They can help a certain amount by phone in terms of medical consultations, or setting up appointments, or doing research. The long distance sibling can also use part of his or her vacation to come and relieve the primary caregiver for awhile, giving the home caregiver a respite. One problem with long distance siblings that

I've read of, as well as heard of from other caregivers, is when they just want to give orders by phone and consider that their contribution. That doesn't work. I know of one family with a half dozen adult offspring who decided that if a sibling is actively involved in a loved one's care, that sibling has a voice and a vote; however, if a sibling doesn't help, then that sibling has no say in the caregiving process.

Family members need to state where they stand on the issue of caregiving for their parent or spouse—what they are personally willing and able to contribute in helping the care recipient. This is not a time for arguments or justification or judgment—just the facts, as Sgt. Joe Friday used to say. Quality of time given can be as important as quantity. When choosing, you might first consider the adage, "Do unto others as you would have them do unto you." Second is a thought about what the afflicted person has done for you. Of course you don't have to get involved in caregiving since life is about free choice. Just be honest. If you don't want to help, just say so. Search your soul and simply state where you stand. You owe that much to yourself, the afflicted family member, and the committed caregiver(s).

If you feel forced into a caregiving situation, to care for someone you never liked, think twice before taking it on. Caregiving and its attendant problems can test you to the limit in the best of relationships; if that were to be complicated by not liking the care recipient at all, then I imagine that a person couldn't do a good job of caregiving. In tough moments, you'll have a shorter fuse, and you may act out your old resentments, resulting in neglect or other abuse of the patient.

If most offspring in a family choose not to help with caregiving, that does not mean they can vote that parent into a nursing home. They can offer an opinion, but the final decision on the patient's future is made by the Health Care Representative or guardian and their assisting physician.

Finally, for those friends and family members who do freely choose to become caregivers, I believe you will experience a sense of personal reward, satisfaction, and love that is beyond comparison. My extensive caregiving experience was for an AD patient, so those are the principal caregivers I have known. I can honestly tell you that I've felt an instant, warm bonding with every one of them I've met—in-person, on the telephone or online. We had shared long periods in the trenches. We were family.

Nursing Homes

People in general appear to be afraid of old age, Alzheimer's disease, nursing homes, and death. Fears of old age, disease, and death are nothing new. Consider the legend of the Buddha from 2,500 years ago. Some of the sages had predicted his future as a holy man, but his father, the king, wanted the boy to be the next monarch after the Father's death. To insure this, the king kept his son in a luxurious palace; made all manner of sensuous pleasure available to him; and ordered that his son not be exposed to the frailties of mankind in the real world. Once, Buddha escaped for a trip outside the palace gates and saw examples of old age, disease, and death. He witnessed the real pain of living, and the experience changed his life forever. He was no longer able to take the selfish and narrow road of complete sensual immersion to escape reality. From that point on, he knew that his destiny was to help mankind first learn to accept all of life and its heartaches, and then find a way to rise above it. Today's reality has some different toys available to escape the sorrows, but the principal dilemma is ultimately the same—facing our own frailties and mortality. Due to the greater longevity of so many people, we now have a relatively new institution to consider—nursing homes. For the Buddha's father, the palace gates served to keep out visions of the disabled and dying; in our day, nursing homes serve that separating function by keeping the disabled and dying elderly inside and away from public view.

*****

Nursing homes are packed with AD patients who have been virtually abandoned by their friends and families. Further, the local agency of the National Council on Aging reviews or interviews all potential residents of nursing homes to make sure the patients are not just being dumped there at government expense for the convenience of the patient's next of kin. I'll never forget that crowded funeral I attended for the deceased AD patient who was a resident at NH #3 for at least four years; and yet I had seen only one of that group of 100 or so attendees visit the patient at the nursing home over the years. That is a lesson in funeral as formality, and perhaps friendship as convenience.

The middle class and poor citizens of America currently have very little hope for decent nursing home care in their disabled old age. The shortage of staff, problems with theft, occasions of abuse and neglect—all these issues, in addition to the immense cost of nursing homes to the people and the federal government, illustrate that we have to find a new solution for the needy aged who face this dismal prospect.

As one example of patient abuse, consider the case of the nurse I mentioned in chapter nine who was fired from NH #3. She had withheld the patients' medications yet had signed the record that she had given them. She had withheld the medications only from the dementia patients—one of them also had cancer—and it took some time for her to be caught. When the demented—to include some mentally ill—patients had been "acting out," as related by another nurse there, doctors were contacted and some medication levels were increased because of it. It's hard to say how long the dementia patients were mistreated by this particular abuse, but it was at least several weeks that the abnormal behaviors had been noted. Even if the dementia patients could verbalize, who would listen to them since the nurse had signed the medication chart as having administered those medications to the patients? Even Mother's physician, who was also the medical director of the facility, seemed indifferent afterward when I thought the facility should pursue some licensing action instead of just firing the nurse. He tried to dismiss the idea with the statement, "These things are going to happen in nursing homes...."

*****

We need a new paradigm or social contract to provide some quality of life for dependent, old people as they approach death. I consider it a gauge of the greatness of a society as to how they treat their old and dying. I believe our society and government are often failing miserably in this respect.

Too many vested interests are making money off of the present nursing home system, and too many people find it convenient to dump their old people there for anyone to be interested in change, until it's their turn of course. Then they will be crying for help, but it will be too late.

*****

I'm reminded of an Alzheimer's patient I met one Christmas night at NH #3. I had finished my visit with Mother, tucked her in, and was on my way to the elevator and home. There was a patient standing near the elevator with a quizzical look. I had seen her once before and assumed she was middle-stage Alzheimer's. She was dressed in nice, casual street clothes, and at a glance no one would suspect that anything was wrong with her. This lady was alone; there were no other patients or staff in sight. As I approached, she said in a bewildered tone, "Excuse me. Can you tell me where I am?"

"Yes, ma'am," I replied. "You're at _____ [name of NH #3]."

"What is that?" She returned.

I could feel where this was going and didn't want to answer, but there was no way out. "It's a nursing home," I answered.

"A nursing home? Why would I be at a nursing home?" She was truly puzzled.

"Someone must have brought you here." I said, as I hoped for both of us that she would stop asking.

"Why would anyone do that to me?" She asked as her bottom lip started shaking in teary sadness.

"I don't know," I answered. "I don't know." I put my arm around her shoulder to comfort her. Soon, an aide came by and walked the lady to her room. That was Christmas night.

*****

We can do better than the system for elderly warehousing that we have now. Maybe nursing homes should be taken out of the free market economy and changed to non-profit status; some already are. Similar to many industries, there are deeply-entrenched financial interests that find the status quo agreeable and pay political figures to keep it that way. Understaffing increases profit levels, and in the corporate world higher profit is the name of the game. However, for the rank-and-file residents who have to suffer through terminal illnesses while other people and businesses profit off of their conditions, we must try more humanitarian solutions. We need to wake up. We are short-sighted at best. As one biblical reference tells us, "Now we see through a glass darkly."

The Value of Family Caregivers

What is currently saving our medical system—at least Medicare and Medicaid—from financial collapse is the free labor provided through the commitment and dedication of family home caregivers. Whether they be family or friends; whether they be motivated by love, duty, or whatever else fuels their service; these are people who make a serious difference in America. They are the unknown soldiers. They're in the trenches and often solitary and isolated. They're not celebrities making the rounds of television appearances and mentioning a disease. These family caregivers give big time as they do the work, day in and day out, *36 hours a day*, day after day, week after week, month after month, and year after year. Many give up their outside jobs. They spend their savings. They spend their retirements. They spend their present lives and their futures. They often sacrifice their health. All this is done to keep their loved ones at home and out of nursing homes for as long as possible. The value of that voluntary labor has been estimated at $257 billion a year,[9] and that estimate is from 2002; hard to tell what it would be now.

Family caregivers are in a class by themselves in the contribution they give to the health and welfare of the nation. Their gift is not only the immense amount of free labor they provide, but the way in which they give it; that is, with body, mind, and soul. These are the most meaningful elements in any real healing and resolution—the bonding agents between caregiver and care recipient that demonstrate the priceless love they share to one degree or another. These qualities and services cannot be purchased at any price in a professional medical system and profit-driven nursing homes. Although love and compassion may be demonstrated to some degree by professional caregivers, those qualities are the controlling motivators and standard currency for family caregivers. Love, compassion, and spiritual bonding are the give and take for family caregivers and their care recipients—the coin of their realm.

*****

In determining the value of medical research in the treatment of Alzheimer's disease, there is a parallel to the relative value of traditional health care services. Medical research is a profession that is helpful in aiming to resolve medical problems that humans face. Like professional caregivers, medical researchers lead regular lives (i.e., with careers, a family life, financial compensation, and a regular work shift). During their work, they contribute to the care and study of human health. Employees in both categories give varying degrees of dedication, love, and compassion in doing their work. Both professional caregivers and medical researchers are of supplementary assistance to the family home caregiver—in the short-term by the care recipient's visits to the clinic; in the long-term by what may be discovered in terms of tools for the caregiver, as well as slowing the onset or progression of the disease, and maybe even finding a cure for AD.

A few other notes on medical research. I spent five years working in the field of aging research as a research assistant. Most of the work was progressive and personally rewarding, and the work environment was very civilized. However, family caregivers often can't wait for the results of medical research in order to get on with the business of caregiving. Researchers commonly work on multi-year projects and then spend more time interpreting their results while family caregivers have to improvise daily on the new challenges that arise in aiding their care recipients. A family caregiver has to think fast and respond to the situation at hand as opposed to waiting for the officially-released medical opinions that might eventually settle in as conventional medical wisdom. For some reason, I'm reminded of the Chinese fortune cookie I got last year; it read, "The philosophy of one century is the common sense of the next." In this case, philosophy represents a method that the caregiver develops to deal with an immediate situation. Some examples can be seen in the tools I mentioned in chapter four, or the additional methods I tried as listed in the chapter on nursing homes. When tools and methods are practiced over time and found to be consistently effective, as well as verified and standardized by medical research, the processes can eventually fall into that category of common sense.

For example, a few years ago a medical research study was conducted on the value of regular exercise for family caregivers in terms of helping them perform their caregiving functions. The results were that physical exercise is beneficial for caregivers in carrying out their caregiving duties. Now, I had known that from the first day I began caregiving eight or nine years earlier. If I had not exercised during all those years of caregiving until the medical research study had verified it, I would probably be dead. Or, if by not exercising I had turned to a harmful substance (e.g., alcohol, tranquilizers, etc.) in order to cope with caregiving; I would be in very bad health. In one scenario I would be dead, and in the other I would be very sick. In either case, I wouldn't have been able to carry out my caregiving commitment. The point is that family caregivers need to be creative and independent-minded in order to deal with the task at hand. It's good to review your caregiving strategy with your physician—especially if it involves exercise for you and the care recipient—but you may find out that you know more about caregiving and its problems than your doctor does. As a caregiver, share what you've learned with your physician, and then he or she may mention that to another caregiver the doctor comes in contact with.

*****

Due to the inappropriate distribution of funds in our bloated medical system, neither money nor personnel are provided to help the family caregivers keep their Alzheimer's patients at home. At least that was my experience. (I've heard recently that some assistance is now available for people who qualify for Medicaid.) It seems the system would rather force patients into a nursing home than aid them in the far more economical and spirit-saving approach of staying at home as long as possible. Again, in the treatment of Alzheimer's disease, family caregivers are in a class by themselves, working 24/7 without financial assistance as opposed to the workaday world of 8/5 with financial compensation.

In this country, respect for a person is often based on how much money the person makes or has accumulated. The practices of true sacrifice and love as they apply to family caregiving do not seem to be recognized as valuable by many Americans in this period of history. That may be one reason so many primary caregivers end up abandoned by other family members when the caregiving issue arises. For many Americans, the phrase "Time is money" has become their standard of conduct. Accordingly, those family members don't want to give up part of their lives to help a needy family member. Fortunately, for the soul of the family and the country—not to mention the benefit of the U.S. economy—millions and millions of family caregivers are willing to make that sacrifice.

So, family caregivers in essence become a family of their own. There is no difference among white, brown, black, red, and yellow-skinned caregivers; nor is there any difference among caregivers of different religions or nationalities; nor is there a difference between caregivers of different genders; nor is there really a difference between the middle class and poor caregiving families except that the poor may have even fewer resources available (depending on their Medicaid eligibility). All family caregivers are brothers and sisters, for these are people who are saddled with the same serious reality—setting their lives aside to take care of disabled loved ones for an often indeterminate period of time.

Few family caregivers ever meet each other or even hear of each other personally. However, they share a common soul and often without knowing it. If they happen to gather in the same area, or find themselves communicating with one another through phone, letter or electronic media, they will find their souls touched and quickly realize that they have arrived home—they are family.

Finally—Me

These past fifteen years have brought a lifetime of ups and downs. While I never expected my caregiving experience to last nearly so long, nor to affect me so long after it was over, I have no regrets. I have found this period to be life-defining, and part of a destiny I had never imagined.

Like many other primary and solitary caregivers, I first experienced anger and resentment with some siblings who abandoned the task at hand and expressed very negative responses. However, I have come to see that matter in an entirely new light. If my siblings had been involved in Mother's care, I would not have gained the satisfaction of completing such a huge task. Nor would I have been able to spend so much time with Mother and help her through the horrors of the disease. Nor would I have been able to experience the degree of unconditional love which grew so much between us during the caregiving process.

In the end, I look back and see the battlefields we crossed, one after another. Through the maze and stress of medical, legal and other institutional issues, as well as the slings and arrows of the ever-ravaging Alzheimer's, we survived and kept our souls intact. All those trying issues were like a series of military campaigns that had to be confronted before we made it through the war. Perhaps it was all just meant to be.

I thank God for the silent help and strength which aided our journey. I thank my wife for her patience and support as she entered our lives only a couple of years after the struggle had begun. I'm grateful that Nancy and Bernice could enjoy each other before the ravages of Alzheimer's dimmed that awareness. I thank my father for having the foresight and knowledge to choose Bernice as his wife, and knowing that she would be the best of mothers for their children.

Most of all, I thank Mother for being a ceaseless teacher and consistent example of how a good life is lived—from the moment my eyes first opened until the moment her eyes last closed. Not that I always followed her example, but without it I would have been completely lost or lived a much poorer life.

The Alzheimer's journey is like living in another galaxy, and each Alzheimer's case is somewhat different from the next, being its own solar system within that galaxy. Fortunately, in our solar system the hard times were augmented by a lot of smiles, laughter, and sparkling eyes. Mother's bright and joyful spirit served as the ever-renewing sun— the fuel to keep me going.

Now that the writing is over, I return to the positive memories of caregiving—those I only carried before the decision to write it all out, before reviewing the aides' notes and my journals and reliving the tough times we had endured as well. In this now positive frame, my mind's eye returns to the early years of caregiving, and a time when we had a respite from the disease. Our common denominator was that of two likeminded, human spirits who were sharing the most simple of human joys—an atmosphere of observing and appreciating nature and the changing seasons.

That fall day we had a period of balmy Indian summer. We sat outside and watched the beautiful leaves drifting lazily down. Mother had just tried to make a bird whistle to fool me as I had previously done to her. She just couldn't get her lips shaped to create a whistle, and the intended whistle sounded more like wind sweeping through a little window. We were both laughing, and she said, "We're having fun, aren't we?" And I completely agreed, "Yes, Mother, we're having fun."

*****

Such are the simple pleasures that make for a peaceful life, and, I believe, a more rewarding and less fearful death. The essence of those moments is unconditional love, acceptance, and joy. If we can absorb those qualities—as did my mother, Bernice Ione Foy Buchanan—then we also have a chance to gain our wings and fly away.

Similar to the fall day mentioned above, last fall brought another day with Indian summer. It was early October—the month I consider the most spectacular weather-wise for perhaps all the country—and time to start putting away the garden. The vegetables were finished though some fruit still remained. The flowers continued brightly and were a visual pleasure until the first freeze.

As I walked among the plants, I noticed the tall Tithonia bushes with their orange blooms. Also called Mexican sunflowers, the Tithonias have beautiful flowers three to four inches in diameter, and they draw bumblebees, hummingbirds, and butterflies. The only activity at the time was a large, bright Monarch butterfly who was dancing in flight from blossom to blossom and bush to bush. She was busy in her work of taking nectar and paid me little heed. In the past, I've touched a couple of Monarchs by stroking the outline of their wings, and they didn't take off.

This butterfly continued her activities as I watched, and then chose to dance off to another bush in the garden, flying within a couple inches of my face en route. Suddenly, the message seemed clear—get back into life; do your work; don't be concerned with what other people think; be self-motivated; and make sure to have some fun every day. That was a lot of information to be spurred by one simple butterfly. However, it was a good reminder to stay alert since teachers and lessons can come in many forms from any direction.

During my long education, I eventually determined that my mother was my greatest teacher. Some of her consistent lessons by example were work hard, stay healthy, be joyful, help others, and love much. I believe that if we can follow that regimen, we will have rewarding lives and an easier transition into the next one. Expanding on a couple of those lessons, I've come to accept that if we live and work with love, then we'll be okay; if we don't, then we're just spinning our wheels at best.

Some years ago, I began to notice the relevance of the people we meet in our lives, and the events we experience. Our interaction with others, and the direct or indirect effect of those meetings, contribute to making our lives like a finely-tuned symphony.

Hopefully, my own case of elderly dependence is a long way off. In the meantime, I return to the workaday world a much richer person with the priceless gems of the joy we shared. My spirit rises, and I will continue to follow the advice of the poet W.H. Auden, "Dance while you can!"

*****

As I began to clear away the mountain of notes, journals, books, research papers, and personal correspondence I accrued during the care-giving process, I came upon the following letter from the secretary of the Masonic Home Kids—the group I mentioned in chapter four that Dad had belonged to and that had invited Mother and me to attend their reunion homecomings after Dad passed away. I had written Betty—the group's secretary—and included a copy of the article about bringing Mother home from NH #2 so that she could share that information with another group who cared so much about Bernice. Betty's letter was dated June 18, 1996—halfway through our caregiving experience. It reads as follows:

> Dear Heydon,
>
> Thank you so much for the warm, loving letter you wrote about your mother. What a beautiful way you have with words. Although I didn't have a chance to know your father as well as I would have liked, I know he would have picked nothing but the best when he got his life mate—"Bernice."
>
> Bernice fit in with Heydon's (Dad's) Home Family so well that we soon forgot she wasn't raised in the home, too. She had a quiet, dignified yet warm manner about her that was unique. She was proof that there is strength in gentleness.
>
> I will publicize her address and hopefully some of us will be able to stop by to see her. I'd like to see that smile of hers even in this stage of her life.
>
> If my sons were able to write so eloquently, I would want them to write what you did when I cease to be able to take care of myself, Heydon. With God's

help, Bernice made you a sensitive, caring individual and
you've been able to tell about it.

> Very sincerely,
>
> Betty   (end of letter)

I'm happy that I found that letter and happy that I was able to
experience the loving camaraderie of that group—the Indiana Masonic
Home Alumni Association. These men and women as children had
faced serious adversity in losing their parents—most of them during the
Depression—and subsequently found strength and understanding
through each other. These phenomenal people not only survived the
Depression and World War II and contributed to the construction of
post-war America; they had the added trauma of being orphans in a very
uncaring world. (My uncle Jim was only four years old and the youngest
of the Buchanan brothers when their father—their last parent—died.)
Yet, all the challenges just made them stronger and very compassionate
with the help of their faith, patriotism, and each other. I believe there
were a couple of hundred "Home kids"—including their spouses—at
the reunions we attended, and they all considered each other full brothers and sisters. They shared a love and mutual acceptance that we all
look for.

A Beautiful Old Age

How shallow we are to dismiss the beauty of the elderly. Those
who age well should be beacons for all of us as we close in on that stage
ourselves. What is aging well? The most positive image given us is that
of a silver-haired pair in good physical form walking hand-in-hand down
the beach as they smile at each other with a full set of sparkling white
teeth; I've seen that picture on ads for vitamins aimed toward seniors.
That's a pretty image and inline with the idea most people would like to
have of themselves—a gracious, sophisticated, loving couple who walk
slowly into the sunset. Yes, it's a nice scene but not really too realistic.
So many old people end up with multiple medical problems, an increasingly narrow view of life, feeling alone and abandoned, and often fearful.
In a term—they lose their smile.

However, there are exceptions, and Bernice was one of them. In
old age, as in earlier life, she set an example of how to transition from

one stage to the next. It's also true that she didn't have to experience the same fear that afflicts so many elderly singles since I was with her all the time; and, as I mentioned early in this writing, she was so appreciative of that.

*****

Bernice was conscious of her look and always took care of herself, always being gracious and loving in appearance and attitude. I don't believe she ever colored a gray or white strand of hair. She aged as God planned it.

To me, the most remarkable sign of maturity was the way she enjoyed life even when the disease was very advanced. During that long final stage of AD, I've seen so many people fall apart physically, mentally, emotionally, and spiritually under the ravages of Alzheimer's; not Bernice. I've see many little old ladies who suddenly come out with a string of profanity that can shock you pretty well; not Bernice. Not one word of profanity, or display of anger or negative attitude at all. Even when few words came out of her, one could see in her face that there was no negative expression. She was really a rare spirit, and everyone I spoke with at the nursing home mentioned it as well. She kept her smile.

The staff loved the photo of us which I've put on the front of this book. And, they also loved the big poster of it which I had placed at the foot of her bed so that when she opened her eyes, she would feel more oriented by seeing me there. I think it helped. How terrifying it must be to feel that steady disintegration of one's memory, one's mind. How vulnerable a person must feel. What anguish the patients must experience as they descend into an abyss and feel the puzzle pieces of their mind moving away from the pattern instead of staying in place.

I read a few years ago about a scientist who received an AD diagnosis. He felt that the medical system or society should help him out in ending his life. He didn't think anyone should have to endure the whole Alzheimer's disintegration. It seems that he was later at home working on some scientific papers, making corrections and notes. Once he finished all that paperwork, he set it aside, picked up a pistol, and shot himself in the head. He left a suicide note that read, "You forced me to do this." He felt that society should have helped him obtain a more peaceful end. Such suicide would be a drastic and lonely road to take. I would have recommended he find a doctor or some trusted advisor who might understand the terror he was going through.

*****

Mother was a different case. She was accepting. She also still had self-consciousness about her appearance which came out in an interesting way. In late stage AD she never thought to look in a mirror and probably wouldn't have remembered what mirrors were anyway. Still, when she laughed with full, open mouth, she was aware that she was missing most of her teeth. (She had had a denture for her upper teeth, but it had disappeared years before on a food tray, and it would have been impossible for her to coordinate with a dentist to construct another one.) She would continue enjoying the laugh but put a hand in front of her mouth to cover it from view.

How interesting it was to see the traits which were so deeply-ingrained, and to notice when each of them began to fall away. Even in very advanced dementia, her manners and consideration for others never slipped; those were based on her love for people, and were so thoroughly embedded in her soul.

When the visiting dentist suggested taking out her few remaining teeth, it made sense for health reasons. At that point, I don't believe Mother noticed the empty spots where those lower front teeth had been. It didn't alter her joyful spirit, and that is what I'm leading up to. The last full laugh we shared, she had no teeth and no inhibitions about that fact. She was Free. At that point, I began to fully realize how beautiful and liberating old age could be if we can move beyond the ego and subsequent vanities, if we *become* spirit.

Her smile then was as joyous, innocent, and sincere as that of a very happy baby—neither of them having teeth or ego or any idea of what those things are. In terms of innocence and beauty, she could have given the Gerber foods baby a run for its money, seriously. There was really no difference in demeanor between the two. The only difference I imagined was that the baby was new to the world, and Bernice was about to leave it. Maybe Mother had an awareness that she was about to shed her cocoon and take on the wings and bright beauty of a butterfly.

May we all keep that joyful and fearless spirit when we reach that stage in life!

2002
Keeping The Faith
Close to the end,
with very advanced
Alzheimer's disease,
yet we could still
share Joy and Love.
Bernice knew
no fear.
Integrity, joy, love,
much work,
much giving,
much sharing—
a good life.

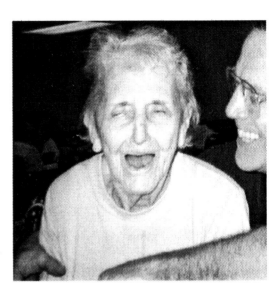

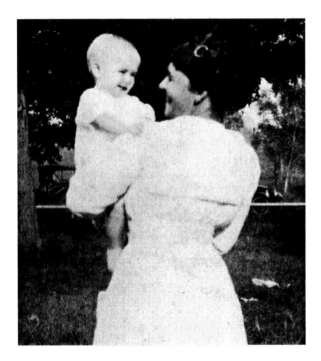

"A little while, and my long-ing shall gather dust and foam for another body. A little while, a moment of rest upon the wind, and another woman shall bear me."

Kahlil Gibran,
The Prophet

Epilogue

Last month I had a dream that was a simple scene and quite beautiful. I was standing on an unpaved, dirt road in the countryside—a road that cut through hay fields that had been mowed close to the ground. There were a couple of people walking in front of me about thirty yards ahead with their backs to me. The person on the right was a short, lean, gray-haired, old woman bent forward about 45 degrees, and the other person was a tall, younger man. With their backs toward me, I couldn't see any faces but I thought I recognized Mother's hair style. She seemed older than when she had passed away, and that was probably due to her posture now having a bow in it; but she was walking again after having been in a wheelchair for the last few years of her life. Then I recognized myself as the man whose arm she was holding for support. As I looked, she turned slowly and stared straight back at me. She was smiling broadly, holding onto my double's arm, and continued walking as she looked back. We had solid eye contact and shared smiles. Then she turned back to face their road, and the two of them started getting farther away. Her support never did turn to face me but kept his eyes on the road and straight ahead. They never stopped walking during that encounter.

I'm not sure what all of that meant. Considering it now, I would say that Mother and her caregiver or support had moved on to another dimension. She was old and bent, but her smile and happiness had not diminished at all, and she was walking again. Her support—the caregiving portion of me—was still helping her, and the two of them were heading over the horizon, maybe going to meet Dad. The still living portion of me was silently saying goodbye to them since I had more life to live before my time came to leave this world.

Offhand, I don't know what role the countryside dirt road and cut hay fields played in the scene. My guess is that it was a hearty, healthy, and natural environment which represented Bernice's life and character as well. Also, there was a more direct reference to that in the earlier-referenced song—

The new mown hay sends all its fragrance
From the fields I used to roam;
When I dream about the moonlight on the Wabash,
Then I long for my Indiana home.

Bernice was a conduit, a liaison, an emissary from that simpler world of yesteryear. Her simplicity, love, joy, sincerity, and heartfelt compassion for everyone represented a combination of characteristics that is not commonly seen. However, I believe that her very existence represented a living example of the inherent Divine potential we all have within ourselves. She was a teacher and loving spirit of the highest order.

Notes

Chapter 2 / Returning Home
1. *The Ballad of Narayama*. Directed by Kisuke Kinoshita. Japan: Shochiku Company Ltd., 1958.
2. Kathryn Spink, *Mother Teresa: A Complete Authorized Biography*. (San Francisco : HarperSanFrancisco, 1997).

Chapter 3 / The Life Well-Lived
1. Ross Lockridge Jr., *Raintree County: which had no boundaries in time and space, where lurked musical and strange names and mythical and lost peoples, and which was itself only a name musical and strange*. (Boston: Houghton Mifflin, 1948).

Chapter 4 / Arriving—Home Is Where The Hearts Are
1. Isabella Alden, *Four Girls at Chautauqua* (Boston: D. Lothrop, 1876).
2. Isabella Alden, *The Chautauqua Girls at Home* (Boston: D. Lothrop, 1877).
3. Isabella Alden, *Four Mothers at Chautauqua* (Boston: D. Lothrop, 1913).

Chapter 5 / Families at the Crossroads
1. William Golding, *Lord of the Flies: a novel*. (New York: Putnam, 1954).
2. Denise Grady, "Nominal Benefits Seen in Drugs for Alzheimer's," New York Times, April 7, 2004, Health section.

Chapter 6 / Forgiveness
1. *Rashomon*. Directed by Akira Kurosawa. Japan: Daiei Company, 1950.

Chapter 8 / Nursing Homes—A Modern, Sad Reality

1. Results of federal study: Robert Pear, "9 of 10 Nursing Homes Lack Adequate Staff, Study Finds," New York Times, February 18, 2002, National section.

2. Bush administration remarks: quoted by Robert Pear, "9 of 10 Nursing Homes Lack Adequate Staff, Study Finds," New York Times, February 18, 2002, National section.

3. Dr. John F. Schnelle, a co-author of the federal report: quoted by Robert Pear, "9 of 10 Nursing Homes Lack Adequate Staff, Study Finds," New York Times, February 18, 2002, National section.

Chapter 9 / Nursing Homes—One, Two, Three

1. Nancy Mace and Peter Rabins, *The 36-hour day: a family guide to caring for persons with Alzheimer's disease, related dementing illnesses, and memory loss in later life.* (Baltimore: Johns Hopkins University Press, 1991)

Chapter 10 / Love and Laughter

1. William James, *The Varieties of Religious Experience* (New York: Modern Library, 1902).

Chapter 11 / A Time to Die

1. Health Care for End-Stage Dementia: Daniel J. Luchins, MD and Patricia Hanrahan, PhD, "What Is Appropriate Health Care for End-Stage Dementia," *Journal of American Geriatrics Society* 1993 Jan; 41(1): 25-30.

2. Edgar Lee Masters, *Spoon River Anthology* (New York: Macmillan, 1914).

3. Stephen B. Oates, *With malice toward none: the life of Abraham Lincoln* (New York: Mentor Books, 1977).

Chapter 12 / Picking Up the Pieces

1. Charles Dickens, *A Tale of Two Cities* (London: Chapman and Hall, 1859).

Chapter 13 / The Future

1. Denise Grady, "Nominal Benefits Seen in Drugs for Alzheimer's," *New York Times*, April 7, 2004, Health section.

2. Lyketsos: quoted by Denise Grady, "Nominal Benefits Seen in Drugs for Alzheimer's," *New York Times*, April 7, 2004, Health section.

3. *THE FORGETTING: A Portrait of Alzheimer's*, first broadcast nationwide on PBS 21 January 2004.

4. David Shenk, *The Forgetting—Alzheimer's: Portrait of an Epidemic* (New York: Doubleday, 2001)

5. Shenk: *THE FORGETTING: A Portrait of Alzheimer's*, first broadcast nationwide on PBS 21 January 2004.

6. Tanzi: *THE FORGETTING: A Portrait of Alzheimer's*, first broadcast nationwide on PBS 21 January 2004.

7. Receiving diagnosis of Alzheimer's disease: S. Holroyd et al., "Attitudes of older adults' on being told the diagnosis of Alzheimer's disease," *Journal of American Geriatrics Society* 1996 Apr; 44(4):400-3.

8. Receiving diagnosis of Alzheimer's disease: Q. Turnbull et al., "Attitudes of elderly subjects toward 'truth telling' for the diagnosis of Alzheimer's disease," *Journal of Geriatric Psychiatry and Neurology* 2003 Jun; 16(2): 90-3.

9. Value of informal caregivers: quoted by National Alliance for Caregiving (www.caregiving.org); P.S. Arno, "Economic Value of Informal Caregiving," Annual Meeting of the American Association of Geriatric Psychiatry, Orlando, FL, February 24, 2002.

ABOUT THE AUTHOR

Born in Alexandria, Virginia, while his father was stationed at the Pentagon, Heydon Buchanan grew up in Florida and Indiana. An army veteran himself, he served overseas in northeastern Thailand in the Army Security Agency. After service, he returned to college and graduated from Indiana University. His final year at the university was spent in a foreign studies program in Lima, Peru—his base for travel by land through most of the South American countries. Returning to the U.S., he worked in the trades of typography and graphic design in New York City and later in Los Angeles.

In early 1991, Heydon joined a higher calling by voluntarily committing to be the primary caregiver for the finest person he's ever known. Without any caregiving or medical training, this loving son relocated to Indianapolis to begin his commitment of the heart. His mother was diagnosed with Alzheimer's disease, and this is the story of their lengthy caregiving journey—a long road with perilous obstacles facing them, yet one on which they maintained a near-constant flow of love and laughter. The experience was life-defining and enriched him spiritually forever.

Following the caregiver period, Heydon worked in medical research on a series of projects studying aging and memory, telemedicine for nursing home care, and early intervention and treatment for dementia patients and support for their caregivers. He resigned from the research work in 2004 because of a lingering and compelling need to tell his caregiving story and help other family caregivers. That led to the writing of this book.

Heydon has spoken to college students en route to becoming social workers and also speaks for the Alzheimer's Association. He has also written articles published in the *Indianapolis Star* on his caregiving journey. An avid organic gardener, he makes great salsa and is an enthusiast of Step Aerobics and Spinning. He and his wife, Nancy, live in Indianapolis.

Printed in the United States
51287LVS00003B/55-69

9 780977 814008